Food Smart

A Nutritional Atlas

Laura Pawlak, Ph.D., R.D.
&
Lisa Turner

Food Smart

A Nutritional Atlas

Copyright © 2001 by Biomed General

2346 Stanwell Drive
Concord, California 94520
USA
Tel: (510) 450-1657
Fax: (510) 450-1336
E-mail: info@biomedbooks.com

Managing Editor: Randy Malat

ISBN 1-893549-03-8

This book is not designed to substitute for professional medical advice. Always consult a medical professional before making major changes in eating habits or use of nutritional supplements.

All brand names and product names used in this book are used for illustrative and educational purposes and are trademarks, registered trademarks, trade names, and copyrighted materials of their respective holders and owners.

Illustrations: Stanley Anderson

About the Authors

Laura Pawlak, Ph.D., R.D., received her master's in nutrition and doctorate in biochemistry from the University of Illinois and did postdoctoral training in immunology at the University of California, San Francisco Medical Center. Dr. Pawlak has been a university instructor, is now in private practice, and is a health and fitness instructor certified by the American College of Sports Medicine. She lectures widely on nutrition and health and is the author of *A Perfect 10: Phyto "New-trients" against Cancers*, *Weight Matters*, *Estrogen Dilemmas*, and *Beyond Estrogen*.

Lisa Turner is a health journalist, author of *Meals that Heal* and *Mostly Macro,* and co-author of *The Enzyme Cure*. Her work appears regularly in *Self, Better Nutrition, Vegetarian Times*, and other publications. Ms. Turner has appeared on local and national television and radio programs, teaches cooking classes, and lectures on food and nutrition. Her educational background includes a master's degree in journalism from the University of Southern California as well as training in nutrition and naturopathy.

About Biomed General

Biomed General is an organization that provides health care professionals with the latest scientific and clinical information. Biomed's live seminars and home-study courses are designed to help health professionals provide better care for their patients. Biomed General operates nationwide in the United States as well as internationally.

For more information about the organization's seminars and home-study courses, please contact:

Biomed General
2346 Stanwell Drive
Concord, California 94520
USA
Tel: (510) 450-1657
Fax: (510) 450-1336
E-mail: info@biomedbooks.com

Table of Contents...

Introduction...

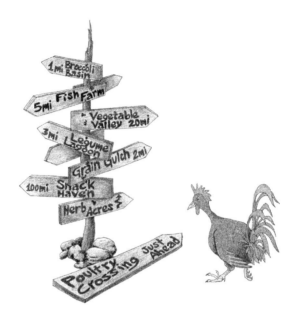

Not so long ago, the idea that food can help prevent disease was a radical view, held mostly by people who grew their own alfalfa sprouts and listened to sitar music. Nowadays, the link between food and health enhancement is so well-established that nutrition issues routinely make the cover of national magazines, and even the most conventional medical professionals are eating their broccoli and cutting down on fat.

It all started in the mid-1980s, with a flurry of findings that demonstrated the irrefutable connection between food and wellness. Since then, study after study has continued to strengthen the evidence linking, on the one hand, specific dietary habits and illness, and on the other, healthy food choices and disease prevention. The findings are impressive:

✗ One in three cancer deaths is directly diet-related; nutrition and dietary factors are believed to contribute to 80 percent of all cancers.[1]

✗ A diet high in fat is a major risk factor for cardiovascular disease, the nation's leading cause of death, while reducing dietary fat can help prevent it.[2]

✗ Eating recommended levels of fiber can reduce risk for a variety of diseases, including cardiovascular disease, diabetes, and certain cancers.[3]

✗ Adequate consumption of fruits and vegetables reduces susceptibility to cancer, cardiovascular disease, and other illnesses.[4]

In other words, we have an extraordinary opportunity to reduce our risk of illness through sound food choices. So extensive and convincing is the evidence that leading health organizations consistently acknowledge the importance of diet as a preventive measure. The National Cancer Institute's "5 A Day for Better Health" program encourages all Americans to eat 5 or more servings of vegetables and fruit daily. The United States Department of Agriculture's (USDA) Dietary Guidelines for Americans advocate a low-fat diet based on whole grains, vegetables, and fruits. The American Heart Association's Eating Plan recommends high consumption of complex carbohydrates while limiting saturated fat and cholesterol.

The implications of what is now known about the food/health link are vast and exciting. In the 1980s and early 1990s, the prevailing position on the health effects of food was founded on fear: poor food choices meant obesity, cancer, and heart disease. The American approach to food consumption focused on what should not be, rather than what was, eaten. As long as we avoided excess quantities of fat, cholesterol, and sodium, we were told, health would proceed along a fairly reliable course, with any illnesses largely the result of genetic misfortune. Not so nowadays. We now know that *a healthy diet is not based solely on what to avoid, but also on what to emphasize.*

As more is revealed about the potent disease-preventive effects of food, especially fruits and vegetables, Americans are moving away from making food choices based on what foods do not contain—fat, sodium, calories—and toward a focus on what they do contain: compounds that can enhance health and wellness. The new way of thinking is that, via what we choose to eat, we may have more control over our health than we thought possible and may be able to prevent even those diseases once considered inevitable. Thus has come a renewed love affair with foods, one infused with a great deal of respect and eagerness.

Specific Healing Compounds in Foods

Above and beyond their energy-sustaining properties, many foods contain components called *phytochemicals* that can offer additional, often extraordinary health benefits. Phytochemicals (*phyto* meaning "plant") are found in whole plant foods—fruits, vegetables, grains, legumes, nuts, seeds—and in less-consumed edibles like licorice, bilberry, and green tea. By the strictest definition, phytochemicals include essential components such as vitamins, minerals, and fiber, but the term is often used to denote lesser-known, nonessential dietary substances.

Phytochemicals have been linked with prevention and treatment of at least four of the leading causes of death in America: cancer, diabetes, heart disease, and hypertension. They are also associated with reduced risk for arthritis, osteoporosis, gastrointestinal disorders, allergies, and immune disorders, among other maladies.[5]

Their mechanisms of action are numerous and diverse. Phytochemicals "may work as antioxidants to offer protection against oxidative damage," says Cyndi Thomson, University of Arizona Clinical Nutrition Research Specialist and spokesperson for the American Dietetic Association. "Some enhance immune function, others alter the expression of different enzymes that play a role in cancer development, still others may act as anticoagulants to prevent plaque formation in the arteries. These mechanisms of action," Thomson adds, "are as numerous as the phytochemicals themselves," and may number "in the hundreds, if not thousands."

The best-known phytochemicals are antioxidant vitamins—vitamins A, C, E, and beta carotene—all associated with lower incidence of cancer and cardiovascular disease. Other vitamins and minerals may have protective effects as well. Folate, for example, is a B vitamin known to reduce the risk of neural tube defects in newborns,[6] not to mention its protective role against coronary heart disease.[7] Calcium can help prevent osteoporosis,[8] while potassium, another essential mineral, plays a role in regulating blood pressure.[9] Vitamin B_6 is helpful in treating premenstrual syndrome.[10] These are but a few examples of "everyday" vitamins and minerals that have proven preventive or healing capabilities.

Five servings of fruits and vegetables daily may provide enough vitamin C to be "beneficial in preventing cancer." So concluded the Food and Nutrition Board of the National Academy of Sciences in April 1999, recommending that the Recommended Dietary Allowance for vitamin C be raised from 60 mg to 100–200 mg daily.[11]

Additionally, research has identified lesser-known phytochemical compounds in everyday foods that have remarkable effects on disease prevention. Some examples:

✗ *Allylic sulfides* in onions and garlic can enhance immune function and stimulate the excretion of carcinogens.[12]

✗ *Isoflavonoids* in tofu and other soy foods can reduce cholesterol levels and help lower the risk of heart disease.[13]

✗ *Isothiocyanates* in brussels sprouts can prevent damage to DNA and may block tumor growth.[14]

✗ *Lutein* and *zeaxanthin* in spinach can decrease the risk of age-related macular degeneration.[15]

✗ *Lycopene,* abundant in tomatoes, can help prevent prostate, lung, and stomach cancer.[16]

✗ *Catechins, tannins, resveratrol,* and other antioxidants in grapes and grape products may help protect against cardiovascular disease[17] and some cancers.[18]

Thousands of phytochemicals in foods have been identified, yet countless more probably remain undiscovered. Similarly, our knowledge of the mechanisms by which these compounds promote health will undoubtedly grow in the coming years. Furthermore, little is known about the amount of phytochemicals needed to achieve health benefits. Animal studies suggest necessary levels, but those levels are hard to extrapolate to human requirements. What we do know is that healing phytochemicals and other health-promoting nutrients exist naturally in a wide variety of whole foods.

Phytochemicals and the Average American Diet

A well-planned diet can probably provide all the necessary nutrients for optimal health. But most Americans do not consume beneficial levels of phytochemicals. In fact, the average American's food choices barely satisfy the most basic nutritional needs and fall far short of safeguarding against disease.

Fruit and vegetable consumption in the U.S. has risen by about 20 percent in the past 25 years.[19] Still, adult Americans are eating on average only 3.1 servings of fruit and vegetables per day,[20] well below the USDA's recommendation of at least 5 servings. Only one of every three Americans meets the minimum vegetable consumption prescribed by the USDA's Dietary Guidelines. Fewer than 20 percent eat enough fruit.[21] These figures may actually be lower if such dubious contestants as potato chips, french fries (which alone account for about 25 percent of all vegetable consumption!), and sweetened fruit drinks are disqualified.[22] The average diet in this country is also very deficient in fiber (11 to 14 grams compared to the recommended 20 to 30 grams).[23]

Beta carotene is a prime example of our sub-par eating habits. The typical American diet provides about 1.5 mg of beta carotene daily, less than one-third of the 5 to 6 milligrams per day recommended by the National Cancer Institute. With a whole-foods diet, it is fairly easy to meet maintenance levels: 6 mg of beta carotene is equivalent to three medium carrots or a handful of dried apricots. Much more challenging, however, is consuming recommended—and health-promoting—levels of beta carotene or other phytochemicals with the average American diet, abundant in processed food but short on fruits and vegetables.

Meanwhile, most Americans still consume an excess of total fat, saturated fat, sodium, and sugar. The percentage of calories from fat has decreased over the last 30 years, but it is still at about 35 percent (30 percent or below is recommended). In fact, Americans are actually eating more fat per capita than 10 years ago.[24] The American Heart Association estimates that reducing average saturated fat consumption from the current 12 to 14 percent of total calories to less than 10 percent can lead to an average 3 to 5 percent drop in coronary heart disease risk.[25] Lowering sodium consumption (from the current 3,000 to 4,000 mg per day to the recommended 2,400 or less) could further reduce the incidence of illness and death from cardiovascular disease.[26]

Not only do Americans continue to make poor nutritional choices—they tend to eat too much. After average calorie intake dropped by nearly 20 percent between 1965 and 1990, by 1995 it had returned to 1965 levels. In 1995, the average American was consuming nearly 500 more calories a day than five years earlier. Increasing consumption of soft drinks, alcohol, and grain products contributed strongly to this trend.[27]

Although the marketplace has been flooded with fat-free products, and the percentage of calories from fat has decreased, sugar consumption is at an all-time high. According to a recent report from the USDA's Human Nutrition Research Center, "Americans daily consume an average of 19 teaspoons of sugar that is added to their foods—by beverage and food processors or by consumers themselves."[28] Too often, Americans choose sugar-rich snack foods and drinks over more nutritious options. The combination of fewer nutrients, added sugar, and extra calories is a formula for increased susceptibility to health problems, including tooth decay, obesity, hypertension, diabetes, heart disease, and cancer.

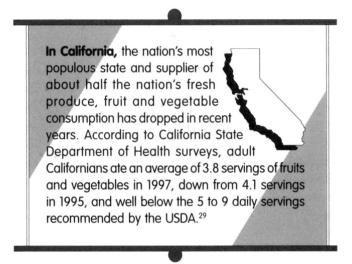

In California, the nation's most populous state and supplier of about half the nation's fresh produce, fruit and vegetable consumption has dropped in recent years. According to California State Department of Health surveys, adult Californians ate an average of 3.8 servings of fruits and vegetables in 1997, down from 4.1 servings in 1995, and well below the 5 to 9 daily servings recommended by the USDA.[29]

From a preventive perspective, so deficient is the American diet that some health professionals and organizations are hinting at various methods of bolstering specific compounds in foods. Children's breakfast cereals, infant formulas, calcium-fortified juices for women, and other food products have long been enhanced with nutrients. Phytochemicals are already finding their way into everyday foods like soft drinks and chips, and the trend toward phytochemical fortification shows no sign of slowing. In the future, bioengineering interests may create foods with varying nutrient levels for specific purposes and at-risk populations. In the meantime, more and more people with sub-optimal diets, often following recommendations from health professionals, have turned to dietary supplements to increase their intake of antioxidant vitamins and other health-enhancing nutrients.

Beyond Broccoli: Supplements and Diet

Because the American diet tends to be limited in whole foods and phytochemicals, some experts say supplementation is critical. According to Stephen L. DeFelice, MD, chairman of the Foundation for Innovation in Medicine in Cranford, New Jersey, the data regarding dietary supplements are clear. "I do believe meals are important, and I would recommend a Mediterranean diet versus a hamburger every day," he says. "But in terms of preventing heart disease and cancer, the research clearly says you need more than you can get in a practical meal." Vitamin E, for example, has been linked to decreased rate of heart attack, but to realize the amounts used in studies, one would have to eat about a cup of corn oil per day.

Numerous scientific papers published in the past five years have shown that increased intake of antioxidants in supplement form can help reduce the risk of cancer and cardiovascular disease. Researchers have consistently concluded that consumption of certain nutrients well above the U.S. Recommended Dietary Allowances (RDAs) may dramatically influence health and disease prevention. "Some supplements are simply more powerful than food," DeFelice says. "I have no religion about it. That's just pure and simple what the research says."

If DeFelice has no religion about it, hundreds of thousands of Americans appear to have decided that if phytochemicals are so powerful, why not just take them in pill form? Sales trends of vitamins and supplements indicate that most Americans seem to have embraced the idea of the vitamin pill as a magic bullet with a fervor that passes fleeting faith and borders on fanaticism. In 1995, Americans spent nearly $2 billion on vitamin and mineral supplements. According to a 1997 Nielsen poll, 72 percent of Americans take supplements on a regular basis. Meanwhile, vitamin sales continue to increase as consumers become more and more aware of the beneficial effect of antioxidant vitamins in particular.

Supplements may indeed help prevent certain ailments and even provide therapeutic benefits, such as slowing the progression of heart disease, cataracts, and perhaps Alzheimer's disease (vitamin E supplementation has been shown to complement conventional treatment of all three illnesses).[30] Yet for every study indicating the potential healing powers gained by supplementing a given nutrient, there are inconclusive or contradictory findings. One well-known study of beta carotene supplementation is an apt example. The study found a *higher* incidence of lung cancer among male Finnish smokers who used beta carotene supplements.[31] It may be that blood levels of beta carotene are merely a marker, indicating the consumption of foods containing other substances that reduce cancer risk. Studies have suggested that beta carotene supplementation will not prevent cancer, unless it is combined with balanced consumption of other antioxidants.[32] Indeed, it may be that the benefits assigned to certain phytochemicals are actually the result of other, yet to be defined constituents.

Much remains unknown about phytochemicals, including levels of efficacy and potential safety issues. Nor has there been adequate identification of the many complex food components that may prevent or treat disease. And although studies have found that supplement taking lowers risk for certain diseases, it may be that supplement users also consume more fruits, vegetables, and other nutrient-dense foods (indeed, they may tend to have healthier lifestyles in general).

Research also suggests that those compounds, when isolated and extracted from food, don't have the same beneficial effects. Perhaps certain food components rely on one another for a synergistic effect, and won't work as well if they're separated from their companion constituents. Moreover, because phytochemicals exist in a fine and precise balance in food, excessive manipulation of one may lead to a tragic imbalance of another. Much research has emphasized the importance of avoiding extremes in nutrient consumption, particularly in the case of isolated nutrients.

Importantly, there are cases in which supplementation is appropriate. For instance, strict vegans (people who consume no animal products, including dairy) may need vitamin B_{12}. As noted, calcium supplementation may be advisable for those at risk of developing osteoporosis. And pregnant women need higher levels of some nutrients, including folate.

There is also growing evidence to support the use of supplements by older adults. Based on studies of the nutritional patterns and needs of people over age 70, researchers at the USDA's Human Research Center on Aging at Tufts University have proposed a modified Food Guide Pyramid for this population—with supplements of calcium, vitamin D, and vitamin B_{12}, as well as eight glasses of water daily, added to current nutritional guidelines.[33] (See page 14.)

Most health advisory agencies, including the USDA, the American Heart Association, and the American Cancer Society, have yet to jump on the supplement bandwagon: they still urge people to fulfill dietary requirements by eating a balanced diet high on whole foods. Overall, it is probably not a good idea to rely on pills for prevention of disease. Until more is known about the kinds and quantities of phytochemicals needed to promote health and reduce disease risk, the best approach echoes mom's advice: eat your vegetables. And fruits, grains, legumes, nuts, and seeds. Specifically, eat at least 5 servings a day of fruits and vegetables—especially dark green, leafy vegetables and red, orange, and yellow fruits and vegetables—along with 6 or more servings of grains and legumes. And don't forget calcium, from dairy or other sources.

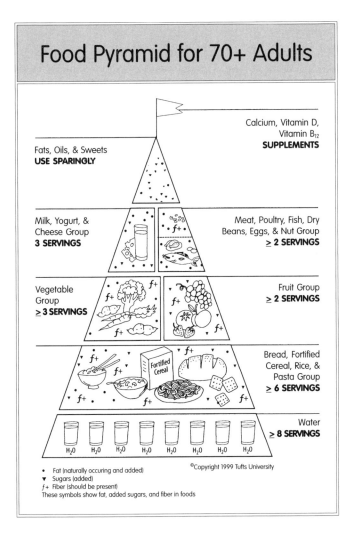

Food Pyramid for 70+ Adults

Calcium, Vitamin D,
Vitamin B₁₂
SUPPLEMENTS

Fats, Oils, & Sweets
USE SPARINGLY

Milk, Yogurt, &
Cheese Group
3 SERVINGS

Meat, Poultry, Fish, Dry
Beans, Eggs, & Nut Group
≥ 2 SERVINGS

Vegetable
Group
≥ 3 SERVINGS

Fruit Group
≥ 2 SERVINGS

Bread, Fortified
Cereal, Rice, &
Pasta Group
≥ 6 SERVINGS

Water
≥ 8 SERVINGS

H₂0 H₂0 H₂0 H₂0 H₂0 H₂0 H₂0 H₂0

• Fat (naturally occuring and added)   ©Copyright 1999 Tufts University
▼ Sugars (added)
ƒ+ Fiber (should be present)
These symbols show fat, added sugars, and fiber in foods

Outsmarting Father Time

Let's not kid ourselves—all of us want to live longer.
Twenty years ago, the primary motives for eating were

social triggers, appeasement of hunger, and immediate sensory gratification. Now, the promise of longevity has been thrown into the mix. While the average life span of Americans is now approaching 80, we are still a long way from our potential. Scientists say the maximum life span for humans is around 115 years. So far, only the Hunzas, a small population of farmers in the Himalayas, have achieved that goal, with reported life spans of 100 to 120 years.[34]

According to current knowledge, a complex combination of factors—such as exercise, lifestyle, and a roll of the genetic dice—determines longevity. As more research comes to light, it seems clear that diet has a great deal to do with how long we can expect to live. Consider the Hunzas. Their diet traditionally consists of grains, fruits, vegetables, and soy, with no meat, eggs, processed fats or oils, sugar, salt, refined flour, alcohol, or caffeine. This nutrient-rich diet appears to be partly responsible for the reported life expectancy, at least as much as a simple, low-stress lifestyle. When the first modern roads were built from the Hunza Valley to China, and processed foodstuffs were imported, chronic diseases began to increase, a phenomenon noted in other primitive cultures that have become Westernized.[35]

In the "developed world," the long average life span of the Japanese is often attributed to dietary factors. The traditional Japanese diet is high in soy products, fruits, vegetables, and fish. Fiber intake is also high, while fat consumption is relatively low. The custom of drinking green tea may also help explain the longer lifespan in Japan. (The Japanese do have an unusually high rate of stomach cancer, a fact that may be explained by their heavy use of salt and salt-preserved foods.)

Below are some of the key dietary factors believed to contribute to longevity.

Calories. Researchers have observed that a reduced-calorie diet can lengthen life expectancy, sometimes dramatically. Restricting calories slows metabolism, reduces body temperature, lowers blood pressure, and may retard developmental processes, including aging. Research animals have been shown to have a one-third increase in life span on a reduced-calorie, nutritionally-adequate diet.[36] If one is restricting calories yet maintaining nutritional adequacy, the diet must necessarily focus on nutrient-dense foods like vegetables, fruits, grains, and beans. On a diet of 1,800 to 2,000 calories a day, there is not much room for nutrient-poor foods high in fats and sugars.

Vegetarianism. A vegetarian diet is also known to increase longevity. Compared to meat eaters, vegetarians tend to get fewer diseases including cancer, cardiovascular disease, and adult-onset diabetes.[37] They have better immunity and lower mortality rates from chronic degenerative diseases.[38] Epidemiological studies have hinted that vegetarians live longer than non-vegetarians by as much as eight years.[39]

Antioxidant protection. A third longevity factor can be addressed with diet. The free-radical theory of aging holds that the body ages in part because free radicals— aggressive and unstable molecules—attack healthy cells, leading to tissue damage and increased susceptibility to disease. Free radicals can be offset with antioxidants like vitamins A, C, and E, beta carotene, selenium, and other antioxidants found in a whole-foods diet.[40]

Oxygen is vital to every cell in the body, but it can also be the cause of degenerative disease. The damaging effects of oxygen can be seen in rusted cars and rancid butter. The same thing happens in our bodies, as part of the normal aging process. Cigarette smoke, environmental pollution, UV light, normal metabolic processes, even excessive exercise, can cause oxidative stress and damage. Fortunately, antioxidant nutrients present in foods can help the body protect itself against this corrosive process.[41]

Even more important than adding years to life is the concept of adding life to years. Living past 100 is a dreary prospect indeed if those additional years are plagued by illness and disease. The exact mechanisms of aging are unknown, nor do researchers agree on whether humans have a genetically-programmed life span. One thing is clear: the years after 50 are marked by an increase in disease, including cardiovascular illness, cancer, neurological degeneration, arthritis, cataracts, and osteoporosis.

By potentially slowing or preventing degenerative disease, a whole-foods diet can enhance overall quality of life, adding life to years as well as years to life. Eating well is about much more than living longer—it's about living *better*.

Given the intimate connection between diet and disease prevention, the grocery store may be where we make the most important decisions about our health.

Getting Smart with Food

As researchers continue to learn more about the causes and treatment of disease, two trends are emerging:

First, *the value of food is measured not so much for its ability to provide sustenance as for its quasi-medicinal properties.* The health-promoting qualities of food are so potent that the grocery store can now be regarded as an emporium for health and wellness, far beyond the first aid and vitamin aisles.

Second, the focus has shifted. *We have become more concerned with what we should eat, rather than what we should not.* The dangers of a high-fat and high-sodium diet have been so widely publicized that the average American knows what to avoid. The question now is, what do we emphasize?

It's a confusing task at times, and many choices must be made, on many levels. We know fruit is healthy. But which fruits are better? What about selecting vegetables: for example, do frozen green beans contain the same phytochemicals as fresh ones? Which foods have the most fiber? And how much fat is in that ground turkey, anyway? Thus the aim of this book: to guide health professionals through the grocery store, aisle by aisle, armed with sufficient facts and information to help consumers make intelligent food choices. Thus, we have designed *Food Smart* as a food-shopping guide. It contains the following:

✘ A rundown of the most common food categories found in grocery stores, and how they fit into a healthy diet.

✘ Highlights on how to select, store, and prepare all the foods needed for health-promoting eating.

✘ Updates of the latest research findings about food and disease prevention.

✘ Data on the specific healing abilities of certain foods.

✘ Details on a vegetarian diet and vegetarian alternatives to meat.

✘ A "shopping cart" of food smart choices.

✘ An appendix listing recommended nutrient consumption levels.

Because the use of food to promote health is a lifelong endeavor, we have put special focus on food choices. No one will stay on an eating plan that prescribes the same foods day after day, year after year. To avoid the broccoli/apples/chicken breast routine, we present numerous healthy alternatives to ordinary food selections. Imagine arugula instead of iceberg lettuce, tropical fruits in place of apples and oranges, bulgur wheat pilaf rather than white rice, and black beans, tofu, or ostrich burgers as an alternative to hamburger.

It's all in here, everything one needs to know to be food smart—to use food choices most likely to contribute to a healthier, longer, better life.

Vegetables...

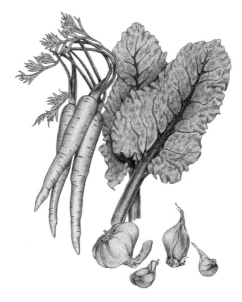

Mom was right about eating our veggies. Averaging only about 25 to 35 calories per serving, fresh vegetables contain more vitamins and minerals per calorie than any other food group. They are free of cholesterol and contain virtually no fat, but they are loaded with fiber. Many vegetables are rich in B vitamins, vitamin C and other antioxidants, calcium, potassium, and iron. Leafy green vegetables are especially high in folic acid. Red, orange, and yellow vegetables are abundant in beta carotene (an antioxidant which converts to vitamin A in the body) and other carotenoids. Vegetables are also packed with various phytochemicals that work in concert with one another to protect against disease.

How Much Is Enough?

Current USDA guidelines call for 3 to 5 servings of vegetables per day. A serving is equivalent to ½ cup of vegetable juice or ½ to 1 cup of cooked or raw vegetables. Some examples:

✗ a bowl of Romaine lettuce
✗ a handful of baby carrots
✗ 4 ounces of carrot juice
✗ a medium artichoke
✗ ½ cup of broccoli
✗ ½ cup of salsa

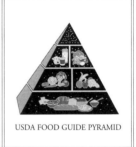

USDA FOOD GUIDE PYRAMID

Overall, given the extraordinary concentration of nutrients and phytochemicals in vegetables, eating a diet high in vegetables is now considered one of the best ways to promote health and reduce disease risk.

Shopping Tips

Fresh vegetables in season and grown locally—or at least in a nearby state—are preferable to those produced farther afield. Produce begins to lose nutrients within a few days after picking. The nearer to home vegetables are grown, the less time it takes to move them from field to store to your home, and the more nutritious they are likely to be.

Chose vegetables that are firm and bright, with a fresh, light scent. Don't buy older vegetables—those that are dried out, shriveled, moldy, cracked, or with a strong aroma; both taste and nutrient value will be compromised. Also avoid buying bruised produce, as it is more likely to contain pesticide residues. Imported produce may be more likely to be treated with pesticides and herbicides not permitted in the United States—another reason why locally- and domestically-grown vegetables (when available) are the most prudent choice. Those concerned about toxins in food may opt for certified organic vegetables. (See "Down on the Farm: A Brief History of Organic Food," pages 37–40.)

Fresh, frozen, and canned. In terms of taste and nutrition, fresh or frozen vegetables are usually preferable to canned varieties. In some cases, vegetables that are frozen immediately retain more nutrients than fresh ones. This is likely if shipping and storage of fresh vegetables takes more than a few days.

Canned vegetables are often mushy and bland, bearing little resemblance to their firm, bright, crisp counterparts. The canning process destroys many water-soluble vitamins, including vitamin C and B vitamins. Yet lost nutrients are added back into some products. In addition, canning does not affect the fiber content of produce. Many canned vegetables are good sources of vitamin A and carotenes (e.g., carrots, spinach, sweet potatoes), folate (beets, peas), and protein. Some canned vegetables may be more nutrient-dense than fresh varieties—depending on the amount of time since harvest and the degree of nutrient-depleting air, light, and heat to which the fresh vegetables have been exposed. Canned foods have a shelf life of about two years.[1]

Several categories of waxes may be used on fresh vegetables to seal in moisture and inhibit molds and fungus. There's also a cosmetic angle: most consumers expect their tomatoes and eggplants to be shiny. The most commonly waxed vegetables are cucumbers, eggplants, peppers, pumpkins, rutabagas, squash, tomatoes, sweet potatoes, and turnips. Fruits are commonly waxed as well. Because waxes may contain chemical fungicides, foods that are waxed should be scrubbed or peeled before eating.

Storage and Preparation

Store fresh vegetables in the refrigerator in loose plastic bags. Greens may be wrapped in a damp paper towel and stored in a plastic bag with holes punched in it. Potatoes and onions may be stored in a cool, dark location. Fresh mushrooms should be stored in a paper bag in the refrigerator.

Wash vegetables just before using. Leafy greens should be immersed completely in a container of cool water to remove dirt. Mushrooms should be wiped with a damp cloth. Root vegetables should be scrubbed with a soft vegetable brush. Waxed vegetables should be scrubbed or peeled before eating.

Garden Variety

Veggies comprise a world of foods and sport a huge variety of healing benefits. Here are some common categories and their nutritional and health-enhancing highlights.

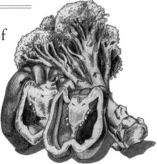

Cruciferous vegetables

Broccoli, cauliflower, broccoflower, red and green cabbage, Chinese (Napa) cabbage, brussels sprouts, radishes, rutabagas, turnips, radicchio, daikon. Collard greens, kale, arugula, and mustard greens are classified as both crucifers and greens.

Cruciferous vegetables contain sulfur compounds which may help lower cholesterol levels and protect against cancer, especially breast cancer. The deep green and red varieties (broccoli, red cabbage, radicchio, greens) are high in cancer-preventive carotenoids.[2] Cruciferous vegetables are also good sources of vitamin C, calcium, magnesium, and potassium. They are high in vitamin K (essential for blood clotting) and excellent sources of fiber.

Peppers

Green, red, yellow, orange, and purple bell peppers, jalapeños, Anaheim chiles, ancho chiles, chipotles, habaneros, Scotch Bonnet peppers, poblano chiles, serrano chiles, banana peppers.

Some Like It Very Hot!!!

Mouth-searing or merely distracting, hot peppers have become the stuff of legend. Some people cannot tolerate them, while others find food bland without hot peppers. They're a good way to liven up low-fat and salt-free dishes, sauces, soups, and stir-fries.

Incidentally, that spicy flavor is more than a gustatory adventure. Capsaicin, the substance that gives peppers their fiery bite, has been shown in some studies to relieve pain, and it may help control blood lipid levels and prevent blood clots.[3]

The Hottest: Orange or red, small and lantern-shaped, *habaneros* (meaning "from Havana") are arguably the hottest peppers of all. Scotch Bonnet peppers are close cousins and about as fiery. Even bold eaters are careful not to use more than a tiny amount, finely chopped, in sauces or other dishes.

The Mildest: Anaheim chiles are similar in taste to bell peppers, but with a bite. They're long and slender, and either green or red. Use them like bell peppers for extra zing—chopped and added to stews and stir-fry dishes, or stuffed and baked.

Handle with care: When chopping hot peppers, be careful not to touch your face or eyes. And don't forget to wash your hands thoroughly afterwards.

Peppers are high in vitamin C, minerals, and fiber. Red and green peppers contain carotenoids, and hot peppers contain a compound called capsaicin, which may help treat pulmonary disorders, lower cholesterol levels, and block pain.[4] In general, the riper (redder) varieties are higher in nutrients than the unripe (greener) varieties.

Greens

Romaine, Bibb, and iceberg lettuce, red and green leaf lettuce, spinach, kale, turnip greens, collard greens, arugula, mustard greens, chicory, Belgian endive, bok choy, dandelion greens, mizuna, escarole, sorrel.

Deep green leafy vegetables are good sources of beta carotene, fiber, calcium, iron, vitamin C, and vitamin K. They also contain folic acid to reduce the risk of heart disease[5] and neural tube birth defects.[6] Spinach is high in lutein, which can prevent or slow macular degeneration.[7]

Healthy as they are, greens do vary nutritionally. For instance, iceberg lettuce can't compare with Romaine in terms of nutrient density.

Mushrooms

Button mushrooms, portobello, morels, cepes, crimini, chanterelles, pom-pom, enoki, shiitake, tree oysters, wood ear, straw. Mushrooms contain B vitamins and potassium and are a source of protein. They also contain compounds that can boost immunity and help protect against cancer.[8] (See "Mushrooms: Suddenly Trendy," pages 35–37.)

Veggin' out...

Can't be bothered with a bowl of spinach? Too tired to chop carrots? Try these fast and simple ways to add more veggies to a daily meal plan.

✗ Use spinach leaves instead of lettuce on sandwiches.

✗ Have carrot or tomato juice instead of coffee for an afternoon break.

✗ Top baked potatoes with salsa instead of sour cream.

✗ Add frozen peas to canned soup before heating.

✗ Make salads creative—add raw corn, water chestnuts, or steamed asparagus.

✗ Sneak peppers, mushrooms, onion, and zucchini into pasta sauces.

✗ Order pizzas with half the cheese and twice the veggies.

✗ Doctor up deli salads with shredded carrots, diced peppers, and chopped celery.

✗ Make a fast lunch at a salad bar, with a plate full of mixed raw vegetables.

✗ Order larger servings of veggie sides with restaurant entrées, and have the vegetable of the day in place of high-fat appetizers.

Root vegetables

Carrots, potatoes, beets, sweet potatoes, yams, turnips, rutabagas, parsnips, burdock, celery root, daikon, fennel, jicama, Jerusalem artichokes. Roots and tubers are good sources of potassium, fiber, and vitamin C.

Orange, yellow, and red roots like carrots, beets, and sweet potatoes have high concentrations of beta carotene and other antioxidants associated with reduction of risk for cancer and heart disease.[9]

Squash

Zucchini, yellow squash, pattypan (scallop) squash, acorn, chayote, spaghetti squash, butternut, banana, blue hubbard, buttercup, pumpkins.

Deep yellow and orange varieties like pumpkin, butternut, and acorn squash are rich in carotenoids. Squash are also good sources of potassium, B vitamins, vitamin C, folic acid, and fiber.

Allium vegetables

Red, yellow, white, Vidalia, Spanish, and pearl onions, shallots, leeks, chives, scallions, garlic, elephant garlic.

These vegetables are great sources of organosulfur compounds (allylic sulfides) found to inhibit clumping of blood platelets, reduce blood cholesterol levels, and lower the risk for certain cancers.[10] They also contain vitamin C, potassium, and trace minerals.

To Everything, There Is a Season

Fresh, seasonal, locally-grown vegetables are usually the best buy, in terms of both money and nutrition. Out-of-season produce has been stored for some time, losing valuable nutrients. Or it may be imported and more expensive. Some vegetables are good all year long: carrots, cabbage, garlic, ginger, mushrooms, onions, potatoes, scallions, and sprouts may be purchased without seasonal considerations. For the rest, there is a season.

January and February

Broccoli, celery, collard greens, fennel, kale, leeks, mustard greens, rutabaga, spinach, winter squash.

March to May

Artichokes, asparagus, broccoli, collard greens, dandelion greens, leeks, mustard greens, peas, new potatoes, sorrel, spinach, watercress.

June to August

Arugula, beets, chard, corn, cucumbers, eggplant, garlic, green beans, kohlrabi, lima beans, okra, peppers, radishes, sorrel, spaghetti squash, yellow squash, pattypan squash, zucchini.

September to December

Arugula, beets, Belgian endive, broccoli, brussels sprouts, cauliflower, celery root, chard, fennel, kale, leeks, mustard greens, parsley, peppers, snow peas, potatoes, pumpkin, rutabaga, sweet potatoes, yams, winter squash.

Fit with Fiber

No question about it: fiber is a crucial component of a healthy lifestyle. The indigestible portion of a plant wall—such as the strings in celery and the skin of corn kernels—fiber helps explain the health-promoting effects of a diet high in vegetables. Fiber aids in digestion and the elimination of waste products. It has a number of other key health benefits as well.

Fiber plays a role in the prevention and treatment of cardiovascular disease through its ability to reduce elevated cholesterol and triglyceride levels and help control blood pressure;[11] there is a correlation between high-fiber diets and low incidence of heart attack.[12] Recent data adds to the evidence that a high-fiber diet helps protect against coronary heart disease.[13]

Fiber is also important in the prevention and treatment of diabetes, due to its role in slowing the absorption of glucose from the small intestine.[14]

High-fiber diets have been linked to reduced risk of breast cancer[15, 16] and prostate cancer, the two leading cancers in the U.S.[17] Studies have consistently shown the importance of fiber in preventing colorectal cancer, this country's fourth most common cancer.[18] Yet recent data have surprised researchers and cast doubts on this conventional wisdom. Findings from the Harvard-based Nurses' Health Study, involving 88,000 women, showed no association between intake of dietary fiber and risk of colorectal cancer.[19] Further research will be needed to determine whether or not fiber provides this important protection.

Nonetheless, the rationale for a high-fiber diet remains strong. In addition to the direct benefits of dietary fiber, high-fiber foods like vegetables, fruits, grains, and legumes are also rich in health-protective phytonutrients. In fact, rates of chronic, degenerative disease are consistently lower in countries with high-fiber diets.

There are two types of fiber—soluble and insoluble:

✘ **Soluble fibers** (gums, mucilages, and pectins) dissolve in water, pass through the digestive system more slowly, and stabilize blood sugar by regulating the absorption of food sugars. Soluble fiber lowers cholesterol levels by increasing bile acid secretions, which in turn breaks down the fats in cholesterol— hence the cardiovascular protection linked to fiber.[20] Carrots and cucumbers are among the vegetables highest in soluble fiber. Many fruits as well as legumes are good soluble fiber sources.

✘ **Insoluble fibers** (cellulose, hemicellulose, and lignin) don't break down in water and have a faster transit time through the intestine. Because they're bulky, they stimulate peristalsis, thus promoting regularity. Insoluble fibers may reduce the risk of intestinal diseases, including cancer, diverticulosis, and hemorrhoids.[21] Insoluble fibers are found in the skins of vegetables and fruit and are also abundant in whole grains.

How much fiber? Current recommendations call for 25 to 30 grams of dietary fiber per day, or 10 to 13 grams per 1,000 calories consumed. But the most recent studies have found that the average American consumes less than half the recommended levels. (Also see "More Fiber Facts," pages 58–59.)

Get your fiber... Vegetables are one of the richest sources of low-calorie fiber. One cup of broccoli contains 5 grams of fiber and only 44 calories. The same amount of fiber from rice adds up to 260 calories. The chart below lists the fiber per 1-cup serving of super-high-fiber veggies.

Carrot	5.2 grams
Corn	6.8 grams
Acorn squash	7.2 grams
Lima beans	6.8 grams
Brussels sprouts	6.6 grams
Sweet potato	6.0 grams
Spinach	4.0 grams
Broccoli	5.0 grams

Yuppie Veggies Spotlight

Bored with broccoli? Had your fill of peas and carrots? Why not try some lesser-known veggies for an adventurous and tasty change of pace. They're dense in nutrients and packed with fiber too.

Fennel is a crunchy, sweetish bulb with an anise-like flavor and a texture like cabbage or celery. Try it roasted with other root vegetables, braised with butter, or chopped raw and tossed into salads.

Arugula, a leafy green that looks a little like dandelion greens, has a pungent, peppery bite. It's great mixed in salads with milder lettuces or chopped and added to soups and stews.

Jicama is a pale brown tuber native to Mexico. It has a crisp white interior with a texture and flavor reminiscent of very mild apples. Cut it into julienne slices and toss with salad for a healthy, crunchy alternative to croutons.

Portobello mushrooms are simply the mature form of crimini mushrooms. The name "portobello" was a marketing ploy to add a sense of glamour and allure. Portobellos have a robust, meaty taste and texture. Slice the stem off and grill the oversized cap whole, or chop and add them to sauces and casseroles.

Jerusalem artichokes, also called sunchokes, are the root of a variety of sunflower plant and aren't related to artichokes at all. They're small and knobby, with a mild, vaguely nutty flavor. Cook them like potatoes—they're especially good baked or boiled—or dice them and add to soups and stews.

Belgian endive is a member of the chicory family, with pale yellowish-green leaves in a slender, cylindrical shape. Its pleasantly bitter flavor and yellowish hue make it a good addition to any salad. The leaves are firm enough to hold up to light braising.

Radicchio, a relative of cabbage, looks like a small red cabbage with thinner, more pliable leaves. It adds color and a slightly bitter flavor to green salads, and can be braised or added to stir-fry dishes.

Broccoflower, another cruciferous vegetable, is what it sounds like: a cross between cauliflower and broccoli. It's shaped like a small cauliflower, with a pale green hue. The flavor is less pungent and slightly sweet. Use it like its namesakes—raw in salads, steamed, in stir-fry dishes, soups, stews, and casseroles.

Mushrooms: Suddenly Trendy

A fondness for fungi has never been the hallmark of American palates. But that's changing. Once hidden in sauces and slipped into stir-fries, mushrooms are popping up as a proud feature on many a plate. And significantly, studies indicate that mushrooms may stimulate the immune system and have other health-enhancing properties.[22]

Now that they're coming out of the dark to add subtle tastes and textures to foods and possibly fortify health while they're at it, it's time to explore fungi options beyond the plain white button mushroom. They may just grow on you.

✗ **Shiitake.** The shiitake mushroom dates back nearly 4,000 years to the Ming Dynasty in China, where it was used not only for royal dishes but also as common medicine. Shiitakes were used to treat respiratory disease, fatigue, and circulatory disorders, and to boost Chi, or essential life force. Shiitakes may play a role in reducing risk for heart disease and cancer.[23]

✗ **Reishi**. Another standard in Asian traditions, reishi mushrooms have been used for thousands of years in both cooking and medicine. In ancient Japanese medicine, the reishi was recognized as an overall strengthening tonic and prized for its ability to ensure eternal youth. Researchers have found that reishi mushrooms can help lower cholesterol and boost immunity.[24]

✗ **Maitake.** In feudal Japan, these feathery fungi were so highly valued they were used like silver as a medium of exchange. Like shiitake and reishi, maitake's main claims to mushroom fame are its anti-tumor and immune-enhancing activities. A compound called D-fraction is the active constituent extracted from maitake; it may inhibit tumor growth and bolster immunity.[25]

✗ **Enoki.** These pale, slender mushrooms with a long, thread-like stem and tiny cap are commonly found in Japanese cooking and as gourmet garnishes. They are traditionally used to stimulate the immune system and prevent ulcers.[26]

✗ **Chanterelle.** Recognized by their brilliant yellow-orange color, these firm, fleshy, French mushrooms are a gourmet mainstay. They're also thought to help prevent night blindness, and research shows that they may guard against certain diseases of the respiratory tract.[27]

✗ **Wood ear.** Also know as tree ear, wood ear mushrooms are dark brown, with a bland taste and jelly-like texture. They are common in Chinese dishes. Wood ears were traditionally used as a stomach tonic in China and applied locally for eye irritations in early European cultures. They may help lower cholesterol levels and boost immunity.[28]

✗ **Oyster.** These soft, pale gray fungi have a delicate flavor and are most often used in Asian dishes. They appear to have modest anti-tumor properties and may help lower cholesterol levels.[29]

✗ **Morel.** Distinctive looking, with a pocked, cone-shaped head, morels have a slightly sweet and pungent taste, and are generally found in gourmet dishes. Traditional Chinese medicine valued the morel for tonifying the intestines and stomach, regulating Chi and reducing phlegm. Like other mushrooms, morels may also have tumor-inhibiting effects.[30]

Down on the Farm: A Brief History of Organic Food

Many, many years ago, eating organic was a simple endeavor. Dinosaurs munched little shoots and grasses of varying colors and flavors. The diet of hunting-gathering peoples was free of synthetically-fertilized roots and seeds and hormone-fed game. Later, when farming entered the picture, farmers stuck seeds in the ground and the seeds grew into food.

With the advent of modern agricultural practices and the use of chemical pesticides, growing practices became more complicated. When enough people decided that they didn't want chemicals with unknown effects on their leafy greens, the modern concept of organics was born. At first, it was viewed as a self-indulgent hobby for extremists. Then came the big Alar scare in 1989. The specter of nasty chemicals in little kids' lunch boxes made the general public take notice of organics. Many people now see organically grown foods as the healthiest choices.

The purpose of organic farming is to create what's called a whole farm system, one that takes into consideration everything from the kinds of seeds used to encouraging biodiversity on the farm—not just in the plants they grow, but also in critters like insects and birds. Organic farmers grow a diverse selection of crops, unlike modern non-organic farming that focuses on one kind of crop, a practice that depletes nutrients in the soil; farmers now "fortify" their fields with added nutrients.

Those crafty producers of food who label products "pesticide free" or "grown without chemical fertilizers" know what they're doing: "pesticide free" or "chemical free" means just that, and nothing more. The verbiage skirts around other issues: herbicides, weed killers, synthetic fertilizers, contaminated soil and air, and other chemicals—not to mention the proactive methods organic farmers use to build a whole farm system.

The only way to be sure produce is organic is to look for the "certified organic" label. There are currently more than 40 independent third-party certification agencies in the United States which make sure that organic foods are in line with currently-accepted standards for growing, storage, transportation, and processing. Those standards are set by states or by the certifying agency.

In early 1999, the USDA announced that it would soon issue guidelines on organic food labeling, which would replace varying state and industry rules. These new national standards will prohibit labeling a food "organic" if it is produced with the help of pesticides, herbicides, preservatives, genetic engineering, irradiation, antibiotics, or hormones.[31]

In the meantime, keep in mind that most grocers carry one of three types of produce:

✗ Conventionally-grown produce is grown with chemical fertilizers and pesticides.

✗ Transitionally-grown produce has been grown without chemical fertilizers and pesticides, but comes from land that's not yet certified for organic production.

✗ Organically-grown produce is certified to be grown without chemical fertilizers or pesticides.

Since the long-term effects of synthetic chemicals aren't known, many people feel safer eating organic or transitional produce. If organic or transitional vegetables aren't available, make sure vegetables are thoroughly washed (scrub the outside of tough vegetables with a soft brush) or peeled.

But don't assume that because produce is organic, it's safe. Outbreaks of foodborne illness have been caused by contaminants in organically-grown produce.

Contamination of any produce can occur during fertilization, shipping, or handling. The bottom line: wash all produce before you eat it.

Just so you know: farmer's market vegetables and fruits aren't necessarily organic. Even farmers who sell what they actually grow may offer produce from local wholesalers to flesh out their selection. If you do shop at farmer's markets, ask the vendors if they grow the food they sell and, if so, what their growing practices are.

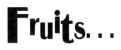

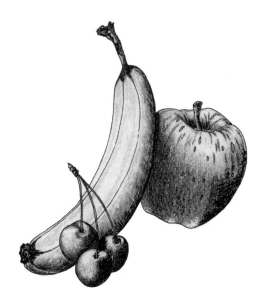

Eve's plucking of the apple in the Garden of Eden forever elevated fruit to the status of fabled food, one that has carried a certain mystique throughout the ages. The word "fruit" comes from the Latin *fructus*, originally meaning "to enjoy"—an apt description. The hundreds of kinds of fruit range from the comfortably familiar apple and orange to exotic tropical varieties like mango and carambola. From a health and nutrition standpoint, few foods can compare.

Fresh fruits are packed with vitamins and minerals, including potassium, folic acid, vitamin C, and beta carotene, with virtually no fat and zero cholesterol. They

How Much Is Enough?

Current USDA guidelines call for 2 to 4 servings of fruit per day. A serving is equivalent to 1 medium-size piece of fresh fruit, ¾ cup of fruit juice, or ¼ cup of dried fruit. Some examples:

✗ ½ cup of strawberries
✗ a big handful of grapes
✗ 1 medium banana
✗ ½ cup of applesauce
✗ a 6-ounce glass of fruit juice
✗ a handful of raisins

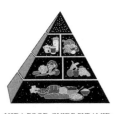

USDA FOOD GUIDE PYRAMID

are also rich in soluble fibers, which can lower cholesterol levels, stabilize blood sugar, and reduce cancer risk.[1, 2] Research has consistently found a significant association between level of fruit consumption and risk for cardiovascular disease[3] and cancer.[4, 5] Other findings indicate that increased fruit consumption helps protect against diabetes, stroke, obesity, diverticulosis, and cataracts.[6] Grapes, oranges, berries, and tomatoes, among other fruits, are especially high in health-promoting phytochemicals. Fruits also offer a source of instant energy: the carbohydrates in fruit are readily digestible.

Shopping Tips

Fruits should be firm and colorful and should smell light and sweet. Avoid those that look bruised, shriveled, molded, cracked, or split. For the best taste and cost savings, purchase fresh fruit in season. Those concerned about the pesticides and herbicides used to treat many fruits may opt for certified organic fruits.

Fresh fruit tends to be more nutritious than canned fruit and is often more flavorful. Frozen fruit also retains more flavor than canned varieties, though its nutrient content is not as high as that of fresh fruit.

Cooking and other processes involved in canning fruit destroy water-soluble vitamins, including vitamin C (the dark color that occurs when fruit is cut and exposed to air is a sign of vitamin C being oxidized and destroyed).[7] Vitamin C is added back into some canned fruits; in fact, some products contain more vitamin C than their fresh counterparts. Canning does not affect the fiber content of fruit. Canned fruits often contain added sugar.

Eating dried fruits—such as raisins and dried apricots—is a convenient way to add fruit to the diet, although some dried fruits are comparatively high in calories.

Fruit juices contain many of the same nutrients as whole fruits, but unless they contain fruit pulp, they are far lower in fiber. For example, an orange contains about 3.7 grams of fiber, compared to about 0.5 grams in an 8-ounce glass of orange juice (fresh-squeezed or from concentrate). (See "Juicy Details," pages 46–47.)

Storage and Safety

Store fresh fruit in the refrigerator if it's very ripe, or unrefrigerated if the room temperature is cool. Grapes and berries should always be refrigerated, as should cut fruit. Never refrigerate bananas.

To ripen fruit faster, place it in a brown paper bag. The natural ethylene gas released during the ripening process converts the starch to sweeter sugars. (This won't work with apples, grapes, berries, or citrus fruits.)

Wash or peel all fresh fruits before eating.

Apples[8]

	Calories	Fiber (grams)	Vitamin C (mg)	Vitamin A (I.U.)
1 medium, with skin	81	3.7	7.9	73
1 medium, skinned	73	2.4	5.1	56
Juice, fresh (1 cup)	117	0.2	2.2	2
Juice, from frozen concentrate (1 cup)	112	0.2	1.4	0
Dried (¼ cup)	52	1.8	0.9	0
Applesauce, sweetened (½ cup)	97	1.5	2.2	14

Join the Fruit-of-the-Month Club

Seasonal fruits grown near home are the best choice whenever they're available. Out-of-season fruit has either spent time in storage or is imported. In either case, it will be less flavorful and more costly than during its season. (Avocados, bananas, kiwi, lemons, limes, and pineapples are generally good year round.) Here's a calendar of fruit highlights:

January through March

Cherimoyas, grapefruit, mandarin oranges, navel oranges, papayas, tangerines, ugli fruit.

April through June

Berries, blood oranges, figs, mangoes, papaya, pears, plums, strawberries, watermelon.

July through September

Apricots, berries, cherries, figs, grapes, mangoes, melons, nectarines, peaches, plums, tomatoes, watermelons.

October through December

Apples, cranberries, figs, grapes, kumquats, mandarin oranges, navel oranges, pears, persimmons, pomegranates, quince, star fruit.

Berry good fruit choice... Sweet and juicy berries are brimming with nutrients, including cancer-preventive carotenoids, and loaded with fiber. One cup of strawberries contains 80 mg of vitamin C and 4 grams of fiber, twice as much as in a slice of whole-wheat bread. Blueberries are high in anthocyanins, compounds that can protect against heart disease.[9] At less than 75 calories per cup (45 for strawberries), berries are great choices for fast and healthy desserts and snacks. Try blackberries, blueberries, currants, elderberries, gooseberries, lingonberries, mulberries, raspberries, strawberries.

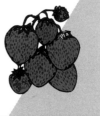

Juicy Details

Juices vary widely in their nutritional content and tastes. Some are the equivalent of liquefied fruit. Others are little more than sweet, colored water. Here are some details:

✗ **Freshly-squeezed or extracted juice** from a juice bar or a home juicer is packed with the most nutrients. (To minimize nutrient loss, drink fresh juice soon after it is squeezed.)

✗ **Fresh frozen juices** are quickly frozen after extraction and retain most of the nutrients and taste.

✗ **Chilled fresh juices**, found in the refrigerated section of the grocery store, are freshly extracted juices that are then packaged for shipping and distribution.

✗ **Frozen juice concentrates** are made by extracting the water from juice and freezing the solid concentrated portion.

✗ **100 percent, canned or bottled juices** may be made from a single fruit or from a blend of fruits to create a certain flavor and level of sweetness. Those made from a single fruit may be sweetened with grape juice.

✗ **Fruit beverages or drinks,** such as Tang® and Snapple®, may contain only a small amount of real juice. These shouldn't be counted as a fruit serving.

Grape juice, packed with antioxidants, may help protect against heart disease[10] and some cancers.[11]

Cranberry juice has been found to be helpful in treating urinary tract infections.[12]

Orange juice is high in folate, another reason to drink it regularly. The latest findings suggest that adults should consume 400 micrograms of folate per day to decrease risk of heart attack, coronary heart disease, and colorectal cancer.[13] Just two glasses of orange juice contain half that amount.

You Say Tomato...

Fruit or vegetable? Actually, tomatoes are a fruit, as are avocados. The botanical classification of a fruit is based on the seed of a plant, 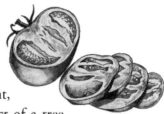 or the reproductive product of a tree or other plant (hence the adjective "fruitful," meaning productive). Whatever the case, the oft-maligned tomato (it was once known as *mala insana,* meaning "unhealthy fruit") is now recognized as an extraordinarily smart food.

There is a strong association between high consumption of tomatoes and tomato-based products and reduced risk for a number of cancers, including cancer of the lung, prostate, stomach, breast, and colon, among other sites.[14] Researchers attribute this protection to lycopene, a relatively rare member of the carotenoid family that is abundant in tomatoes. This potent antioxidant is also thought to boost immunity and maintain mental and physical functioning during the aging process.

The research suggests that cooking and processing tomatoes does not diminish these beneficial effects. Moreover, tomato sauce and tomato paste are highly-concentrated sources of lycopene. Be aware, however, that fats, sugars, and sodium are often added to tomatoes in the canning process. Homemade tomato sauce may be the best bet: tomatoes cooked with a little oil seem to be the most effective way to deliver lycopene.[15, 16]

Genetically-engineered tomatoes containing five times more lycopene than usual are now available in some parts of the country.

Tomatoes[17]

	Calories	Fiber (grams)	Lycopene (mg)	Vitamin C*	Sodium (mg)
Fresh (1 medium)	26	1.4	5	40%	11
Sauce (½ cup)	30	2	17	20%	640
Canned (½ cup)	25	1	11	15%	220
Canned, no salt added (½ cup)	35	2	11	20%	20
Paste (2 tbsp)	25	0.5	8	10%	80
Sun-dried (1 piece)	27	0.2	NA	5%	47
Juice (8 ounces)	50	2	20	20%	620

*Percentage of Recommended Daily Value based on a 2,000 calorie diet.

Fruitful Endeavors

Here are some fast and easy ways to add fruit to daily meal plans:

✗ Keep single-serving cans of 100 percent orange juice or grapefruit juice on hand for a fast serving of fruit.

✗ Take a bag of grapes or sweet cherries to the movies to munch on instead of popcorn.

✗ Freeze grapes, bananas, or chunks of mango for healthy dessert treats.

✗ Whirl frozen berries and banana in a blender with a little milk or yogurt.

✗ Try dried cranberries, papaya, mango slices, apricots, and raisins as nutritious alternatives to candy.

✗ Keep fruit salads interesting by combining fresh and dried fruit, then top with shredded, unsweetened coconut and a spoonful of vanilla yogurt.

✗ Add chopped apples, raisins, or diced pineapple to coleslaw, chicken salad, or tuna salad.

✗ Toss clementine oranges (small, portable, and pre-packaged in their own easy-to-peel skin) in a purse or briefcase for a fast snack on the go.

✗ Try tropical fruits for an exotic change of taste.

✗ Use 100 percent fruit juice and fruit preserves as the base for fat-free salad dressing and marinades. Mix 1 part juice, 1 part preserves, and 2 parts vinegar.

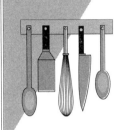

Hot Fruit! Baked fruit makes a delicious and healthy dessert.

To bake bananas, first preheat oven to 350° F. Place a banana (skin included) in a baking dish and bake until thoroughly blackened (takes about 20 minutes). Remove from oven, slice open, and spoon into a dish. Sprinkle with brown sugar, vanilla, and raisins, and serve hot.

To bake peaches, apples, or pears, preheat oven to 375° F. Core apples, cut pears in half lengthwise and remove seeds, and cut peach in half and remove pit. Place fruit in a baking dish, sprinkle with chopped pecans, vanilla, and raisins. Add a little apple juice to the baking dish, cover with foil, and bake until just tender (takes about 25 minutes). Serve hot with a sprinkle of granola and cinnamon.

Foreign Fruits

Not so long ago, few exotic fruits, other than bananas and pineapple, were available to U.S. shoppers this side of the tropics. But that has changed: exotic fruits are now on hand at supermarkets and produce markets across the country. Like fruits in general, exotic fruits are packed with nutrients and fiber and have zero fat and cholesterol. Remember that the red, orange, and yellow varieties (such as mango, papaya, pomegranate) are loaded with beta carotene to neutralize free radicals and lessen the effects of aging.[18]

Asian pear, or Oriental pear, is shaped like an apple, but with a juicy crispness and light sweetness that more closely resembles a pear.

Carambola, also known as star fruit, is a glossy yellow fruit with a light, fragrant taste reminiscent of plums.

Cherimoya, or custard apple, has a firm, greenish exterior with large scales, with a sweet, creamy, custard-like interior.

Kumquats look like small, oval-shaped citrus fruits and taste like an orange. They're eaten whole, rind and all.

Mangoes, when ripe, are intensely sweet and fragrant, with a taste similar to very ripe peaches and a smooth, almost creamy texture. They should be fairly soft, with a reddish yellow skin. The variety known as "Manila mangoes," yellow when ripe, have a smaller pit and are especially flavorful.

Papaya, often confused with mango, has a very different taste. Shaped like avocados, with smooth, yellowish green skin, papayas are lighter tasting than mangoes, and the texture is more like a melon.

Persimmons have a smooth, thin, shiny skin, and the interior is fragrant and sweet, tasting something like a very ripe plum. They should be a deep, rich orange, and very soft—if not completely ripe, persimmons have an unpleasant, mouth-puckering quality.

Pomegranates have a tough, leathery skin in a rosy hue. The inside is filled with edible seeds surrounded by a juicy, deep red pulp that's sweet and light.

Ugli fruits are about the size and shape of a grapefruit, with a thick, loose, green skin. They taste like a cross between a grapefruit and a mandarin orange.

Dried fruits have an intense flavor and sweetness that makes them ideal for a fast snack, instead of sugary treats. They add instant flavor to many dishes: dried apples add interest to chicken or tuna salad, and a handful of dried cranberries or raisins turns a plain bowl of rice into a special treat. Incidentally, dried fruits are packed with nutrients, especially potassium and antioxidant vitamins. Look for dried apples, apricots, bananas, currants, cherries, cranberries, dates, figs, mangoes, peaches, pears, papayas, pineapples, prunes, and raisins.

Grains...

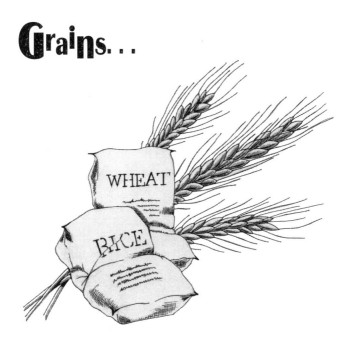

Long ago, when early families began planting the seeds of grasses (what we call wheat), they settled together to protect their crops, instead of wandering from berry bush to grassy field. Based around the cultivation of grains, these earliest permanent settlements grew into what we now know as civilization.

Grains provide the base of the USDA Food Guide Pyramid and are the most widely consumed food group. Every culture has its uses for this irreplaceable staple, from Asian rice to Italian pasta to Latin American corn tortillas.

Grains are good sources of vitamin E and B vitamins. One B vitamin, folate, regulates blood levels of the amino

How Much Is Enough?

The USDA recommends 6 to 11 servings of grains per day, in the form of breads, cereals, pasta, or rice. A serving is equivalent to 1 slice of bread, 1 ounce of ready-to-eat cereal, or ½ cup of cooked cereal, grains, or pasta. Some other examples:

✗ ½ cup of oatmeal or rice
✗ a small bowl of pasta
✗ ½ corn on the cob
✗ 1 slice of whole-wheat bread
✗ ½ bagel

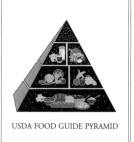

USDA FOOD GUIDE PYRAMID

acid homocysteine to decrease the risk of atherosclerosis, heart attack, and stroke.[1] Whole grains are rich in fiber, another protector against atherogenic as well as carcinogenic processes. In addition, grains contain phytic acid, also known as IP-6, a phytochemical which can prevent the formation of free radicals[2] and may protect against breast, colon, and liver cancers.[3, 4]

Many people do not realize that grains contain a fair amount of protein, which can be combined with beans, lentils, or other plant sources of protein to form complete proteins.

Shopping, Storage, and Cooking Tips

Because most of the nutrients and fiber are contained in the outer layers of grains, it's best to select whole-grain products. Seek out different grains in cereals, pasta, crackers, bread, and other baked goods. Whole grains can often be purchased in bulk at natural food stores. Look for intact kernels that aren't broken, scratched, or damaged.

Store grains in a cool, dark, dry area, in a sealed glass or plastic container.

Grains can be prepared in a variety of ways: boiled or pressure cooked as a side dish, used in casseroles, soups, stews, and salads, ground into flours and made into breads and other baked goods, formed into pasta or cereals—the possibilities are nearly endless.

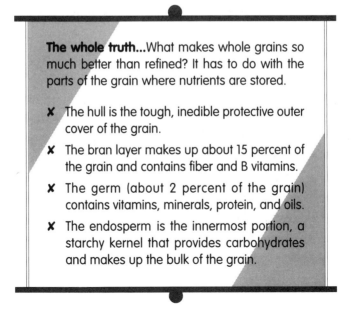

The whole truth... What makes whole grains so much better than refined? It has to do with the parts of the grain where nutrients are stored.

✗ The hull is the tough, inedible protective outer cover of the grain.

✗ The bran layer makes up about 15 percent of the grain and contains fiber and B vitamins.

✗ The germ (about 2 percent of the grain) contains vitamins, minerals, protein, and oils.

✗ The endosperm is the innermost portion, a starchy kernel that provides carbohydrates and makes up the bulk of the grain.

More Fiber Facts

Fiber, non-digestible material from plants, is one of the greatest nutritional virtues of grain. Whole grains are good sources of both soluble and insoluble fibers. As noted in "Fit with Fiber" (See pages 31–33), fiber plays an important role in protecting against heart disease and heart attack by helping control blood cholesterol levels, triglyceride counts, and blood pressure. It also helps in the prevention and treatment of diabetes as well as in the lowering risk for some cancers, including breast and prostate cancer.

> Researchers have observed a 37-percent reduction in the incidence of coronary heart disease for every 5 gram increase in consumption of soluble fiber from cereals.[5]

Fiber aids in digestion and helps prevent constipation—and fiber from wheat or oat bran is more effective at increasing fecal bulk than fruits, vegetables, or purified cellulose fiber.[6]

Recommendations for dietary fiber intake for adults generally fall in the range of 20 to 35 grams per day, or 10 to 13 grams of fiber per 1,000 calories. One serving of most whole grains contains 2 to 5 grams of fiber.

Introducing high quantities of fiber into a low-fiber diet can cause gastric distress, including cramping and in some cases constipation. Add fiber gradually, and increase water intake.

Grains[7]
(½-cup serving)

	Calories	Protein (grams)	Fiber (grams)	Folate (mcg)
Rice, brown, long grain	108	2.5	1.8	4
Rice, white, long grain	103	2.1	0.3	46
Bulgur wheat	76	2.8	4.1	17
Barley, pearled	97	1.8	3.0	13
Oats	73	3.0	2.0	5
Oats, instant, fortified	69	2.9	2.0	100
Buckwheat groats	78	2.9	2.2	12

Waves of Grain

Wheat is the most familiar grain, but lots of other options exist, each with its own unique nutritional aspects.

Barley has two inedible outer hulls that are removed in the milling process. The remaining outer layer, called the aleurone layer, is rich in protein, fiber, and B vitamins. Because the aleurone layer is often removed in a process called "pearling," look for whole hulled barley instead of pearled barley for higher nutrition. *Combine 1 part barley and 2 parts water, bring to a boil, reduce heat, and simmer for 1½ hours.*

Buckwheat has a distinctive tan seed with three corners. Toasted, it's called kasha. Buckwheat has more of the essential amino acid lysine than any other cereal grain. Cook it as a whole-grain breakfast cereal or side dish, or use in flour form for pancakes and baking. *Combine 1 cup buckwheat with 2 cups water, bring to a boil, reduce heat, and simmer for 20 to 25 minutes.*

Corn is the only common grain that contains vitamin A. It's low in the essential amino acids lysine and tryptophan, but eaten with beans it provides all of the dietary amino acids needed to form a complete protein. Blue corn has a higher nutritional value, with more protein, potassium, and manganese than yellow corn, and adds a wonderful color to pancakes and baked goods. Cornmeal is used to make polenta and in baking. Look for the stone-ground variety, which retains the nutritious germ. *Add 1 part cornmeal to 4 parts boiling water, reduce heat and simmer for 25 to 30 minutes.*

Millet is a tiny, round seed with a pale yellow color, has a higher protein content than wheat, and is completely gluten-free. *Combine 1 part millet and 2½ parts water, bring to a boil, reduce heat and simmer for 1½ hours.*

Oats are a good source of cholesterol-lowering soluble fibers. They have a hard, inedible hull that must be removed in milling, leaving the edible bran and germ (called groats). Oats are in two basic forms: rolled oats are used to make oatmeal, and more finely rolled oats are called quick cooking oats. Instant oatmeal is precooked rolled oats. Steel cut (Scotch) oats are cut into small pieces and have a fuller flavor, but take longer

Corn[8]

	Calories	Protein (grams)	Fiber (grams)	Folate (mcg)	Vitamin A (RE*)	Sodium (mg)
Sweet, yellow (½ cup)	89	2.7	2.3	38	18	14
Sweet, yellow, canned (½ cup)	66	2.1	1.6	40	0	265
Sweet, white, canned (½ cup)	66	2.1	1.6	40	0	265
Sweet, yellow, cob, frozen (½ cup)	76	2.6	2.3	25	17	3
Sweet, yellow, canned, cream (½ cup)	92	2.2	1.5	57	13	365
Corn tortillas (2)	115	2.9	2.7	59	0	6
Corn bread (1 piece)	173	4.4	0	42	35	428
Popcorn, unsalted (1 cup)	30	1.0	1.2	2	2	0.3
Corn chips (1 ounce)	152	1.9	1.4	6	3	179

*micrograms Retinol Equivalents

to cook than rolled oats. *Add 1 part rolled oats to 2 parts boiling water, reduce heat and cook over low heat for 15 minutes (5 minutes for quick oats).*

Rice in its whole form (brown rice) is a good source of B vitamins and other vitamins and minerals. White rice is rice from which the nutritious bran and germ layers have been removed. Rice comes in short, medium, and long-grain varieties that differ mainly in taste and texture. Shorter grains tend to be chewier and sweeter, while longer grains are lighter and fluffier. Aromatic rices, like basmati, jasmine, and popcorn rice, are different varieties of long-grain rice known for their fragrant aroma and taste. *Combine 1 part brown rice and 2 parts water, bring to a boil, reduce heat and simmer for 45 minutes.*

Rye is high in the essential amino acid lysine, and can be cooked alone or added to soups, breads, or salads. *Combine 1 part rye and 4 parts water, bring to a boil, reduce heat and simmer for 1½ hours.*

Wheat has two modern varieties—winter wheat and spring wheat—and three basic strains: hard, used in bread baking; soft, used in pastries; and durum, used for making pasta. Cracked wheat is used in Middle Eastern cooking, and makes an excellent rice substitute. Bulgur wheat is cracked wheat that has been parboiled to reduce cooking time. Refined wheat, in the form of white flour, is stripped of its nutritionally-rich bran and germ layers, then bleached to make it whiter. Couscous is made from refined durum wheat and looks like tiny grains (a whole-wheat variety is sometimes available). Farina is a refined cereal made from ground and sifted

Flour power... One of the best ways to get grains into any diet is with baked goods. Nearly all grains are available in flour form for baking: a good way to break out of the whole-wheat rut and try different grains. Not all grains can be substituted for wheat flour in baking, since the texture, taste, and gluten content vary dramatically. (Gluten is responsible for the elastic quality of bread dough and for the shape and texture of baked goods.) Best bets for baking: barley, oat, rye, kamut, spelt, triticale. Other flours that have little or no gluten—such as buckwheat, cornmeal, chickpea, millet, quinoa, rice flour—can be combined with a gluten flour for the best breads, or used alone with increased leavening.

wheat. *Combine 1 part cracked wheat or bulgur and 2 parts water, bring to a boil, reduce heat and simmer for 20 minutes.*

Wild rice isn't a rice at all, but rather the seed of a water grass native to the northern United States. Nor is "wild" rice wild—most is grown in commercial rice paddies, and has an inferior taste and texture. Look for true wild rice, available in natural food and specialty stores. Wild rice is usually combined with long-grain brown rice or other rices. *Combine 1 part wild rice and 3 parts water, bring to a boil, reduce heat and simmer for 1 hour.*

Using Your Noodle

Noodles are a fast-cooking, convenient way to add a variety of grains to your diet. They have a fair amount of protein and very little fat: a 1-cup serving of most pasta contains about 200 calories, with 6 to 8 grams of protein and less than 1 gram of fat. It's the sauces and toppings that make pasta pack on the pounds. (To limit fat, opt for fat-free marinara sauces, or top pasta with a tiny bit of olive oil and a handful of fresh herbs.)

The defining factor in pasta, besides the shape, is the type of flour used. Durum wheat, the most common pasta grain, is a very hard wheat with a high gluten content, for a resilient dough that holds its shape in boiling water. Semolina wheat is durum flour with the bran and germ removed. Whole-wheat pasta made from durum wheat is the best nutritional choice—it contains all the vitamins and minerals that occur naturally in the whole grain, and three times more fiber than refined wheat pasta made from semolina. Other noodle choices:

Egg noodles. Made from flour, water, and eggs, they have a deep yellow color and richer flavor. Egg noodles are higher in calories and contain cholesterol.

Colored pastas. Some wheat pastas are colored with vegetables like spinach or beets to add color and eye appeal—but with absolutely no nutritional impact.

Fresh pasta. The nutritional lineup is the same as for dried pasta, the cooking time is much shorter (about 3 minutes), and the taste is either far superior or deplorable depending on how well-made the fresh pasta is.

The breakfast cereal aisle: proceed with caution... Grains are great food, and a bowl of 100 percent whole-grain flakes is a fast, convenient, and healthy way to start the day. Unfortunately, after grains are rendered into typical breakfast cereals, they can be inimical to a healthy diet.

Most cereals use refined grains, so they're fortified with synthetic vitamins and minerals, and sometimes fiber, to up the nutritional content and replace what was stripped off in the refining process. Moreover, most cereals contain a hefty dose of refined sugar—some as much as 15 grams per serving or 30 percent of total volume (compared to the less than 5 percent sucrose in many cereals made by cooking whole grains). Healthy-sounding names can mislead, by focusing on the bran or fruit in high-sugar cereals. So-called "natural" cereals are often no better: many are loaded with sugar, often appearing under the guise of corn syrup or fructose.[9]

Even granola has taken a beating. Traditionally made with oats, whole grains, nuts, fruits and honey, today's granola is usually made with refined white sugar, hydrogenated oils, salt, and preservatives. Compared to a bran cereal, for instance, it is likely to be highly caloric, burdened with fat, and lower in fiber.

Finding cereals made with whole grains can require careful label reading. Look for whole-grain cereals (oats and bran cereals usually qualify, for example). Cereals labeled "Heart Healthy" are good options.

Wheat-free pastas. Designed for people with wheat allergies, these are nice choices for a change. Try brown rice pasta, quinoa, corn, kamut, and spelt. (Kamut and spelt do contain gluten, but they're usually tolerated by people with wheat allergies.)

Asian pastas. Made with lower-gluten wheat, Asian noodles are more tender and porous than American pastas. The rice flour, mung bean starch, buckwheat, mugwort, wild mountain yam, and other kinds of flour used in various Asian noodles gives them a unique flavor and texture—try them for a nice change of pace. They can be served in the traditional Asian fashion—in light, savory broths—or used with nearly any pasta sauce.

Four-for-a-dollar ramen noodle packets, although convenient for a fast meal, are made from white flour deep-fried in partially hydrogenated vegetable oil. They contain up to 10 grams of fat (4 or 5 grams of saturated fat) and at least 800 mg of sodium per serving, as well as MSG, additives, and preservatives.

Ancient Grains: The New Staff of Life

They call wheat the staff of life, but for people with wheat sensitivities, it can be a troublesome food. After years of hybridization, modern wheat isn't the same food our ancestors ate. The gluten content (gluten is part of the protein in grains that makes bread dough rise well)

Pastas[10]
(1-cup serving; about 56 grams)

	Calories	Protein (grams)	Fat (grams)	Fiber (mg)	Folate*	Sodium (mg)
Egg noodles	220	10	2.5	2	30%	15
Spaghetti	200	7	0	2	25%	0
Spaghetti, whole-wheat	190–210	6–10	0	3–6	NA	0
Fettucini	200	7	0	2	30%	0
Linguini, fresh	160	7	1.5	1	NA	15
Ravioli, cheese, fresh	200	9.5	6	2	NA	220
Rainbow rotini	190	7	1	2	25%	10
Soba noodles	200	8	0	2	NA	70
Rice stick noodles	300	8	0	NA	NA	310
Instant ramen style noodles	240	6	10	2	NA	1,020

*Percentage of Recommended Daily Value based on 2,000 calorie diet

is much higher, thus increasing the likelihood of an allergic reaction. People who are allergic to wheat aren't usually sensitive to the wheat itself, but to its higher gluten content.

Enter "ancient grains," low-gluten grains less likely to produce an allergic reaction. Another plus: most are 40 to 50 percent higher in protein than wheat. Look for them in health food stores and in specialty breads, crackers, chips, and cereals, or serve them like rice or oatmeal as a breakfast porridge or side dish.

Kamut. Originally cultivated in Egypt more than 4,000 years ago, the name itself comes from the ancient Egyptian word for "wheat." Kamut does contain gluten, but most people with wheat allergies or sensitivities can tolerate it. It's a better choice even for people who aren't specifically allergic to wheat, since it's more digestible.

Kamut flour can be substituted for wheat flour in most recipes, but is too dense for light yeasted breads. Kamut berries can be sprouted and used in salads, and the large, chewy grains are good in casseroles. *Combine 1 part kamut with 3 parts water. Bring to a boil, reduce heat and simmer 35 to 45 minutes.*

Spelt. This grain was first used around 5,000 BC in Persia. It has a tough outer husk that keeps the grain's nutrients from oxidizing and protects the kernel from pollutants. Even though it does contain gluten, it seems to be tolerated by most wheat-sensitive people.

Spelt can be substituted for wheat flour in most recipes, and is especially good for cookies, muffins, and quick breads. Use it in soups and stews to add texture, much like barley. *Combine 1 part spelt with 3 parts water. Bring to a boil, reduce heat and simmer 1½ hours.*

Quinoa. Pronounced "keen-wa," this so-called grain is in fact the fruit of a weedy plant long cultivated in the Andes mountain region, mostly in Peru and Bolivia. Because it's completely gluten-free, quinoa is appropriate for wheat-free and gluten-free diets.

In baking, quinoa flour must be combined with a gluten-containing flour for yeast breads. Quinoa grains can be used instead of rice or millet in soups, salads, casseroles, and main dishes. (The outer part of quinoa is coated with saponin, a sticky, bitter-tasting substance that acts as a natural insect repellent but can aggravate digestion. Rinse quinoa well in cool water before cooking to remove the saponin.) *Combine 1 part quinoa with 2 parts water. Bring to a boil, reduce heat and simmer 20 to 25 minutes.*

Amaranth. Originating in South America and Central America and a staple food for the Aztecs, amaranth is actually a seed from a broad leaf plant. Practically gluten-free, it is a good alternative to wheat.

In baked goods, amaranth is combined in small amounts with other flours for a lighter flavor and textures. Arrowroot or potato starch can lighten baked goods made with amaranth. The seeds may be popped like popcorn, or added to baked goods for flavor and crunch. (Boiled amaranth congeals as it cools, so it must be eaten right away.) *Combine 1 part amaranth with 3 parts water. Bring to a boil, reduce heat and simmer 20 to 25 minutes.*

Triticale. A hybrid of durum wheat and rye, this grain takes its name from the botanical names of wheat (*Triticum*) and rye (*Secale*). It's very low in gluten and is tolerated well by many people with wheat allergies.

Triticale may be substituted for wheat flour in cookies, cakes, and quick breads. For yeast breads, it should be combined with a gluten-containing flour. Use the berries for sprouting, or like rice in casseroles and side dishes. *Combine 1 part triticale with 2 parts water. Bring to a boil, reduce heat and simmer 2 hours.*

Breads...

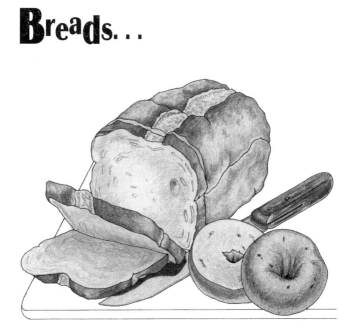

Few foods are as universal in their use and appeal, and as varied in selection, as breads. From sweet muffins to hearty rye bread, French rolls to Mexican tortillas and Indian chapati, breads have a place in every cuisine and at every meal. The varieties are nearly countless, from pre-sliced sandwich bread, bagels and crisp breads, to whole loaves hot from the supermarket's bakery.

Breads—especially whole-grain varieties—are good sources of a number of vitamins, minerals, and fiber. They also contain protein—2 grams or more per slice. Many types of bread are fortified with extra nutrients. Chosen wisely, breads can be nutritious components of meals as well as healthy snacks.

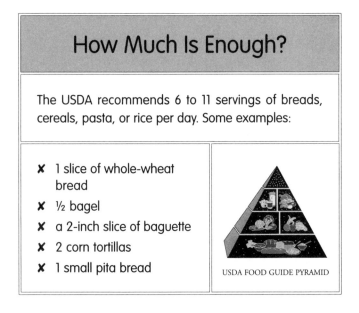

How Much Is Enough?

The USDA recommends 6 to 11 servings of breads, cereals, pasta, or rice per day. Some examples:

✗ 1 slice of whole-wheat bread
✗ ½ bagel
✗ a 2-inch slice of baguette
✗ 2 corn tortillas
✗ 1 small pita bread

USDA FOOD GUIDE PYRAMID

Shopping Tips

Whole-grain breads are the most nutritious choice. They typically have at least three times the fiber content of breads made from refined flour (such as white bread and egg bread). They also tend to be higher in complex carbohydrates, B vitamins, vitamin E, folic acid, iron, zinc, and a number of other minerals.

Whole-grain breads vary in fiber content, so check labels. Those with 2 grams per slice are considered high-fiber. Some breads, especially those made with specialty flours, are higher in protein as well. Whole-grain breads typically contain about 70 to 80 calories per slice. Reduced-calorie varieties are available.

Storage

Store breads in a dark place like a bread box, wrapped in a clean towel or in a perforated plastic bag, at room temperature—refrigerating bread makes it go stale faster. Tortillas, chapatis, and other quick breads should be refrigerated, however, since they mold quickly. Crisp breads such as matzo should be stored in a tightly sealed plastic bag.

Smaller, thinner loaves like baguettes dry out faster, so they should be eaten within a day. Stale bread can be freshened up by steaming it or warming it in the oven.

To Steam: Cut the bread into thick pieces and place it in a vegetable steamer over boiling water, uncovered, for 2 to 3 minutes.

To Bake: Preheat oven to 350° F. Sprinkle stale bread with water, wrap it loosely in foil, and bake it for 10 minutes.

Finding Phytos in Bread

If it's the whole-grain variety, your morning toast may be rich in phytochemicals. A few highlights:

- ✗ **Fiber** can reduce the risk of some cancers[1, 2, 3] and heart disease.[4]

- ✗ **Vitamin E** is a potent antioxidant believed to play a role in promoting arterial health and possibly protecting against cancer.[5]

Breads[6]
(based on 25- to 26-gram slice or as indicated)

	Calories	Fiber (grams)	Protein (grams)	Fat (grams)
Bagel, onion (½)	122	1.0	4.7	0.7
Cracked wheat	65	1.4	2.2	2.0
Egg	70	0.6	2.4	1.5
English muffin (½)	67	0.8	2.2	0.5
English muffin, whole-wheat (½)	58	1.9	2.5	0.6
French	69	0.8	2.2	0.8
Matzo, plain (1 ounce)	112	0.9	2.9	0.4
Mixed-grain	65	1.7	2.6	1.0
Oat bran	60	1.2	2.2	1.1
Pita, white (4 inch)	77	0.6	2.5	0.3
Pita, whole-wheat	74	2.1	2.7	1.0
Pumpernickel	65	2.2	2.2	0.8
Rye	63	1.5	2.0	0.8
Tortilla, corn (medium)	58	1.4	1.5	0.3
Tortilla, flour (6 inch)	104	1.1	2.8	2.3
Wheat	65	1.1	2.3	1.0
White	67	0.6	2.0	0.9
Whole-wheat	69	1.9	2.7	1.2

✗ **Phytic acid** prevents the formation of free radicals, decreases cholesterol and triglycerides, and helps eliminate heavy metals from the body.[7] It may also protect against cancer by binding excess iron in the intestine.[8]

✗ **Folic acid**, a B vitamin, regulates blood levels of the amino acid homocysteine to decrease the risk of atherosclerosis, stroke, and heart attack.[9]

Adding a serving of fresh fruit to whole-grain toast will give an even bigger phyto boost.

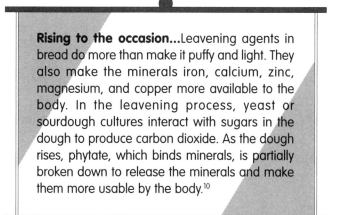

Rising to the occasion... Leavening agents in bread do more than make it puffy and light. They also make the minerals iron, calcium, zinc, magnesium, and copper more available to the body. In the leavening process, yeast or sourdough cultures interact with sugars in the dough to produce carbon dioxide. As the dough rises, phytate, which binds minerals, is partially broken down to release the minerals and make them more usable by the body.[10]

A Loaf of Bread, a Jug of Wine

As noted, whole-grain breads are the most nutritionally dense. Among them, the nutritional lineup is similar. The main differences are shape and texture. Choosing

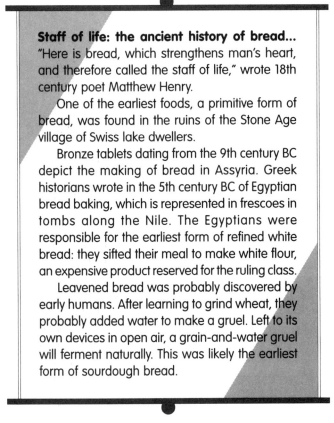

Staff of life: the ancient history of bread...
"Here is bread, which strengthens man's heart, and therefore called the staff of life," wrote 18th century poet Matthew Henry.

One of the earliest foods, a primitive form of bread, was found in the ruins of the Stone Age village of Swiss lake dwellers.

Bronze tablets dating from the 9th century BC depict the making of bread in Assyria. Greek historians wrote in the 5th century BC of Egyptian bread baking, which is represented in frescoes in tombs along the Nile. The Egyptians were responsible for the earliest form of refined white bread: they sifted their meal to make white flour, an expensive product reserved for the ruling class.

Leavened bread was probably discovered by early humans. After learning to grind wheat, they probably added water to make a gruel. Left to its own devices in open air, a grain-and-water gruel will ferment naturally. This was likely the earliest form of sourdough bread.

among whole-grain bread options depends mostly on personal preference.

High-fiber breads are enriched with wheat bran, oat bran, pea fiber, soy fiber, or seeds.

Sprouted-grain breads are made from sprouted wheat or other grains. They have a higher protein content and are thought to be easier to digest, since sprouting converts some of the complex starches to simpler sugars.

Rye bread is usually made with a combination of rye and wheat (typically white wheat flour, not whole wheat). One-hundred percent rye breads are wonderfully moist and dense, and are higher in fiber.

Kamut and spelt breads, made with "ancient grains," were initially formulated for people with allergies. The gluten in kamut and spelt is usually tolerated by people who are sensitive to wheat or wheat gluten. They're usually denser and drier than wheat breads. (See "Ancient Grains: The New Staff of Life," pages 66–70.)

Rice breads contain no gluten, so they're good substitutes for people with severe wheat allergies, but they're gritty and porous, and generally less flavorful. They're usually in the freezer section.

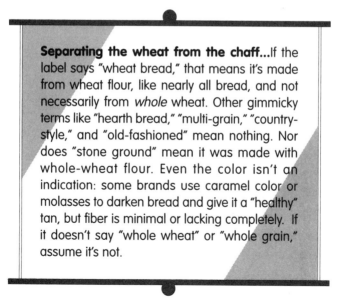

Separating the wheat from the chaff... If the label says "wheat bread," that means it's made from wheat flour, like nearly all bread, and not necessarily from *whole* wheat. Other gimmicky terms like "hearth bread," "multi-grain," "country-style," and "old-fashioned" mean nothing. Nor does "stone ground" mean it was made with whole-wheat flour. Even the color isn't an indication: some brands use caramel color or molasses to darken bread and give it a "healthy" tan, but fiber is minimal or lacking completely. If it doesn't say "whole wheat" or "whole grain," assume it's not.

Pita bread, also called Bible bread, was traditionally used in the Middle East instead of utensils to scoop up food. It comes in refined- and whole-grain varieties.

Bagels can be a fast, healthy breakfast choice, if they're made from whole grains and served with a little jam. Even without cream cheese, the calorie count can be hefty—most are 200 to 300 calories per bagel.

Less than wonder-ful... Puffy white breads have been the mainstay of many a school lunch box, but bread has come a long way since the bran revolution of the early 1980s. White breads have fallen into disfavor with some people: they're mere nutritional shadows of breads made with whole wheat and other whole grains. White bread is made with refined white flour that has been stripped of its fiber and most of its nutrients, then re-enriched with synthetic vitamins. Varieties usually contain saturated fats and trans-fats, refined sugars, artificial dough conditioners, preservatives, and coloring. Check labels. A few newly-available varieties contain added iron, calcium, and fiber. Better yet, stick to whole-grain breads.

Tortillas are unleavened breads made from corn or wheat, and briefly cooked on a hot griddle. Check labels for fats, and choose those made with unhydrogenated oils. Find them refrigerated or in the specialty foods section. Be aware that, compared to corn tortillas, those made of flour have about double the calories and at least two more grams of fat. Significantly, corn tortillas are rich in calcium—45 mg of per 6-inch corn tortilla—at least twice the calcium content of most breads. This is because the corn has been soaked in calcium oxide, also known as limestone or slaked lime, to remove the coating of the kernel.

Chapatis are traditional flat breads made without leavening, traditionally served with curries and other Indian dishes. The whole-grain varieties have more fiber. Find them in the refrigerated section.

Dairy & Eggs...

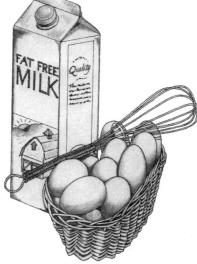

Americans love milk and other dairy foods, part of world cuisine since time immemorial. Cows, goats, sheep, and yaks have been raised for their milk for thousands of years. Traditionally, until the advent of modern dairies and processing plants, milking, butter making, and cheese making have been done by women. The word "dairy" comes from the Middle English *dey*, a female servant.

Milk, cheese, and other dairy foods are rich in protein, vitamins A and D, and minerals, especially calcium. Since dairy is a complete protein, it's considered a good alternative to meat—although some dairy foods made with whole milk are just as high in saturated fat.

How Much Is Enough?

Current USDA guidelines call for 2 or more servings of dairy products a day for adults over 24 and children 2 to 10 years of age; 3 to 4 servings a day for those ages 11 to 24 and for women who are pregnant or breastfeeding. A serving of dairy is equivalent to 1 cup of milk or yogurt, 1 ounce of cheese, or ½ cup of cottage cheese. Some examples:

✗ a 1-inch cube of cheese
✗ an 8-ounce container of yogurt
✗ a small mound of cottage cheese
✗ 8 ounces of skim milk

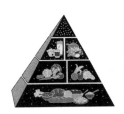

USDA FOOD GUIDE PYRAMID

Shopping Tips

Reduced-fat and fat-free versions of dairy products are the healthiest options. Check labels, however: a reduced-fat cheese may still derive up to 65 percent of its calories from fat. Fat-free cheeses made with skim milk and whey are available, but they're usually rubbery and bland, retaining little resemblance to real cheese. Cheese is often high in sodium, a concern for sodium watchers. Lower-sodium versions are available—again, with some compromise in flavor.

Milk may be packaged in plastic, paper, or glass. Paper cartons are best, because they block most of the damaging light rays from the sun, which can deteriorate vitamins and change the flavor of milk.

Storage and Cooking

Refrigerate dairy products promptly after buying, and store them at 39° F or less. Milk and most other dairy products cannot be sold after a certain date indicated on the package. Typically, they spoil a few days after that date. Keep milk and other dairy foods out of direct sunlight.

Soft cheeses, such as ricotta and Brie, should be eaten within 4 or 5 days of purchase. Hard cheeses can be refrigerated for several weeks. As a rule, the harder the cheese, the longer it will keep.

Serve cheese at room temperature for the best flavor. Cook over low to medium heat—high temperatures will make it rubbery and hard.

A Dairy Diary

A stunning array of dairy products is available in most supermarkets. Here's a rundown of leading dairy products.

Reduced-fat milk. Low-fat milk has a fat content ranging from 0.5 to 2 percent of total calories. Skim milk is milk that has had as much fat removed as possible; a tiny fraction may remain. Both are healthier versions of whole milk, with the same amounts of calcium and protein.

Acidophilus milk is cultured with *Lactobacillus acidophilus*, a friendly bacteria that makes it easier to digest. Unlike yogurt, it is not fermented and has a light, sweet flavor. Use it like regular milk.

Flavored milk contains flavorings, colors, sweeteners, stabilizers, and other additives. The fat content varies, and fat-free versions are a better choice, but they're still high in calories, sugar, and artificial ingredients.

Evaporated milk is made by heating milk, adding stabilizers to firm up the proteins, and concentrating the product in a vacuum. Evaporated skim milk contains less than 0.5 percent fat. Both versions are highly processed and have a thin, weak appearance and lifeless flavor. Use for baking, or in a pinch.

Buttermilk was originally a by-product of the butter-churning process. It is now made by adding cultured bacteria to low-fat or skim milk and incubating the mixture for about 12 hours. During the fermentation process, the bacteria convert some of the lactose in the milk into lactic acid, lending it a distinctive, tangy taste. The thick, rich consistency makes it seem high in fat, but fat content of buttermilk is less than 0.5 percent. Use it in baked goods for a lighter, more tender consistency (buttermilk reacts with baking soda in baking recipes to form carbon dioxide, adding a little leavening boost).

Non-fat dry milk is pasteurized skim milk with all the water removed to make a dry powder that's reconstituted by adding water. Most of the nutrients are retained during processing. It's good for traveling, since it carries without spoiling. Otherwise, best used in cooking, rather than straight up. Non-fat dry milk can be added to some foods—such as yogurt and mashed potatoes—to increase protein and calcium content.

Milk Options[1]
(8-ounce serving)

	Calories	Fat (grams)	Saturated fat (grams)	Calcium (grams)
Milk, whole	150	8.2	5.1	291
Milk, 2% fat	137	4.9	3.0	297
Milk, 1% fat	102	2.6	1.6	300
Milk, fat-free	85	0.4	0.3	302
Buttermilk, low-fat	99	2.2	0.2	36
Milk, chocolate	208	8.5	5.3	280
Milk, goat	168	10.1	6.5	326
Milk, goat, low-fat	90	2.5	1.5	250
Milk, canned, evaporated	339	19	11.6	657
Milk, dry, whole	158	8.5	5.4	291
Milk, dry, non-fat	108	0.2	0.1	377
Cream, half and half	315	28	17	254
Kefir, 2% fat	240	4.5	3.0	300

Goat's milk is a little higher in fat than whole milk, but the fat globules in goat's milk are smaller than those in cow's milk, making digestion easier. Use it just like cow's milk.

Cream is the fat layer of whole milk, containing at least 18 percent fat. Half and-half is a mixture of cream and whole milk which contains between 10.5 and 18 percent fat. Since most of the fats in cream are saturated, use it sparingly, if at all. Best uses: a spoonful of half-and-half in coffee or tea or a dollop of whipped cream on desserts.

Butter is made from cream that has been churned. Butter has a high fat and cholesterol content—one tablespoon contains 36 milligrams of cholesterol. Use it sparingly—spread thinly on bread and muffins and combined with olive oil for cooking. For baking, butter works better than margarine.

Margarine was originally made from lard as a less costly alternative to butter. Now it's typically made from "hydrogenated" vegetable oils and is free of cholesterol. In the hydrogenation process, hydrogen is added to oils to turn them solid, creating compounds called trans-fatty acids, which have been implicated in increased risk for heart disease.[2] Softer margarines contain less trans-fatty acids. Margarine without hydrogenated oils and trans-fats is sometimes available. There is evidence that such products have a more favorable effect on blood cholesterol levels and cardiovascular risk compared to either margarines with trans-fats or butter.[3]

Take Control® (made from soy) and Benecol® (made from wood pulp) are new, specialized margarines developed as cholesterol-lowering "nutraceuticals."

Like butter, margarine should be used in small amounts. It may be useful in strict vegetarian or kosher diets. (Also see "Fats and Oils," pages 161–170.)

"Light" butter is made by combining butter and margarine or hydrogenated oil for a lower calorie count. It combines the worst of both worlds—saturated fat from butter, dangerous trans-fatty acids from margarine. Butter is preferable.

Sour cream has been pasteurized and cultured with *Streptococcus lactobacillus* bacteria, and contains at least 18 percent fat. It's a marvelous treat stirred into hearty stews or as a topping for berries. Just use sparingly—a teaspoon at a time. Reduced-fat varieties exist, though they are less tasty. Yogurt and cottage cheese are reasonable substitutes.

Cottage cheese is made by inoculating milk with lactic acid bacteria, then combining it with cream and salt. Dry curd cottage cheese from low-fat and fat-free milk is lower in fat and sodium, but is also shorter on taste. (Cottage cheese may contain artificial ingredients and preservatives, so read the labels if this is a concern.) Combine cottage cheese with fresh fruit or chopped tomatoes and herbs, or puree it in a blender until very smooth and use instead of cream or sour cream in spreads, dips, and salad dressings.

As the world churns... It's thought that butter was "discovered" by nomadic peoples and shepherds who carried whole milk in animal skin containers on their journeys. When they opened their pouches after a long, bumpy trip, they found that the milk had turned into a rich, creamy mass now known as butter and a liquid we call buttermilk.

This is what happened in those animal skin pouches: as the camels bumped along across the desert, air was incorporated into the whole milk. Membranes which keep the globules of fat apart in the milk were softened and then broken, and the fat began to coagulate. Lecithin from the ruptured membranes helped the fat globules mass together until they came together in a creamy solid, leaving sweet, light buttermilk behind.

Cheese, Please

Making cheese is a true art, rendering plain old milk into the complex foodstuff we know and love. In the simplest of terms, cheese is made by adding a curdling agent to milk to coagulate the solids, pressing out the remaining liquid (whey), cooking the solids (curds), pressing them into shapes, and aging the resulting cheese until it's ready to eat. The actual process is, of course, more complex, with a number of factors that account for the variations in the taste and texture of different cheeses.

Being dairy careful... Since milk is so highly perishable, it has to be handled with a certain amount of care. Most states require pasteurization to kill harmful bacteria. Some purists believe raw milk is better: in the heating process, vitamins are destroyed, minerals like calcium are compromised, and enzymes that make milk easier to digest are killed. Even so, raw milk in modern times probably isn't a safe choice. To make milk safe to drink, it typically goes through three specific processes:

✗ **Pasteurization**. Milk is heated to 161° F or higher for 15 seconds, to destroy any harmful bacteria, molds, yeasts, and other pathogens. Pasteurization also dramatically extends the shelf life of milk.

✗ **Ultra-pasteurization**. Milk is heated at 280° F for 2 to 4 seconds to ensure the complete destruction of all microorganisms. It is then cooled rapidly to 45° F and sealed in sterile containers. Ultra-pasteurization is used primarily with cream products.

✗ **Homogenization**. Milk is sprayed through a nozzle at very high pressure against a hard, flat surface to break up fat globules. The smaller particles of fat are able to remain suspended evenly throughout the product, creating a uniform consistency.

Lost nutrients (and then some) are added back to processed milk products.

The kind of milk used (cow, goat, sheep) will obviously affect the taste, as will ripening conditions like temperature, humidity, and length of time cured. Most cheeses are white or pale yellow. Blue cheese gets its color from special molds. Orange cheeses are colored with vegetable colorings derived from beta carotene or annatto seed (also called achiote seed, with a rusty, reddish color, from the seed of the annatto tree).

Fresh cheeses (cream cheese, farmer's cheese, fresh mozzarella, mascarpone, kefir, hoop cheese) are uncured and the most perishable. They can be eaten right away.

Soft cheeses (Brie, Camembert, Muenster, Port Salut) are ripened briefly and have a very high water content—usually about 50 percent.

Semi-hard cheeses (mozzarella, Gouda, Monterey Jack, provolone, string cheese, kasseri, Edam, Bel Paese, Havarti) have a moisture content below 40 percent.

Most cheeses contain 20 to 30 percent protein per total calories. Some, like mozzarella and especially Parmesan, are higher than average in protein. Cottage cheese has a very high protein content, about 70 percent of total calories.

Hard cheeses (cheddar, feta, Swiss, Emmenthaler, Gruyère, Jarlsberg, aged Gouda) have a very low moisture content. These cheeses are further classed depending on the length of time they're aged. Mild cheeses are cured 2 to 3 months, mellow cheese is cured 4 to 7 months, and sharp cheese is cured 8 months or longer. (Incidentally, among hard cheeses, cheddar is unusually high in fat. It derives about 75 percent of total calories from fat, equal to the fat ratio of Brie and some other softer, seemingly-oilier cheeses.)

Selected Cheeses[4]
(1-ounce slice)

	Calories	Protein (grams)	Total fat (grams)	Saturated fat (grams)	Calcium (mg)
American	106	6.3	8.9	5.6	174
Brie	95	5.9	7.8	4.9	52
Cheddar	114	7.1	9.4	6.0	204
Cream	99	2.2	9.9	6.2	23
Feta	75	4.0	6.0	4.2	140
Monterey	106	6.9	8.6	5.4	211
Mozzarella, whole milk	80	5.5	6.1	3.7	147
Mozzarella, part skim	72	6.9	4.5	2.9	183
Muenster	104	6.6	8.5	5.4	203
Parmesan, grated	129	11.8	8.5	5.4	390
Ricotta, part skim	39	3.2	2.2	1.4	77
Swiss	107	8.1	7.8	5.0	272

Blue cheeses (Gorgonzola, Roquefort, Stilton, Danish Bleu) are soft cheeses that have been inoculated with *Penicillium* molds, creating the characteristic blue-green veining.

Grating cheeses (Parmesan, Parmigiano-Reggiano, Asiago, Pecorino Romano) are very hard and dry, with a longer aging process and the least water content.

> Parmesan cheese has the highest calcium content of any cheese. Swiss cheese is also unusually high in calcium.

Washed rind cheeses (Limburger, Chaumes, Morbier) are cured in a brine of water, salt, and spices, and aged for several months in very high humidity to keep the cheese moist and flavorful.

Pasteurized processed cheeses are made by combining several soft cheeses into a smooth mixture. Pasteurized processed cheese food is a combination of pasteurized processed cheese, whey, cream, milk, or buttermilk. These cheeses usually contain artificial flavors, colors, preservatives, sugar, and lots of salt. Not a good cheese choice.

A Cultural Thing

Fermented milk products like yogurt and kefir have a long and exotic history, both gastronomically and medically. In one telling tale from yogurt lore, legend

Wary of dairy? Lactose intolerance... Lactose, the primary carbohydrate in milk, accounts for more than half of the total non-fat solids in milk. Many people (ranging from 20 percent of Caucasian Americans to 80 percent of Asian Americans and Native Americans)[5] lack sufficient lactase, the enzyme that breaks lactose down into its component sugars. As a result, they are unable to digest milk products properly. This condition is known as lactose intolerance. Its incidence increases with age. Symptoms include stomach cramps, bloating, gas, increased mucus production, and diarrhea.[6]

Lactose-digesting enzyme products, in tablets and liquid form, can make dairy easier to digest, and lactase-fortified milk products can help as well. So can consuming only small amounts of dairy products at a time. Goat milk, raw dairy products, yogurt, and other cultured foods like kefir and buttermilk are generally better tolerated. Aged cheese and cottage cheese contain less lactose and are easier to digest.

has it that in the 16th century, King François I of France summoned a young Turkish doctor to cure his chronic diarrhea. The doctor came equipped with sheep and his secret recipe for yogurt, and the king was soon well on his way to recovery.

Around the turn of the 20th century, Nobel-prize winning biologist Elie Metchnikoff suggested that lactobacilli—strains of friendly bacteria found in cultured milk products—could ease certain gastrointestinal ailments. Researchers have pinpointed a variety of health benefits from the friendly bacteria in yogurt and kefir, including treatment of gastrointestinal disorders,[7] enhanced immune function,[8] and possible cholesterol-lowering[9] and anti-cancer effects.[10]

Yogurt is made from milk that has been fermented by *Streptococcus thermophilus* and *Lactobacillus bulgaricus*—the bacteria responsible for the health benefits of yogurt—using specific times and temperatures. Look for the terms "living yogurt cultures" or "contains active cultures" on yogurt labels—to make sure you're not buying dead bugs. Combine yogurt with honey and fruit, or use in place of sour cream. Incidentally, yogurt is sometimes used as a "probiotic"— eaten to prevent yeast infections by women taking antibiotics.

Kefir, a thick and creamy, slightly bubbly dairy drink, was perhaps the first health beverage, its reputation going back thousands of years—its name derives from the Turkish word meaning "good feeling." Kefir is made by fermenting milk with a complex mixture of bacteria, including various species of lactobacilli. The compounds produced by these friendly organisms lend kefir its characteristic fizzy and sweet/tangy flavor. Use kefir in breakfast smoothies for a fresh, different taste, or as the base for salad dressings.

Yogurt and Cottage Cheese[11]
(½-cup serving)

	Calories	Fat (grams)	Saturated fat (grams)	Calcium (mg)
Yogurt, plain, whole milk	95	4.0	2.5	200
Yogurt, plain, low-fat	70	1.3	0.8	200
Yogurt, plain, non-fat	60	0	0	225
Yogurt, fruit, low-fat	115	1.3	0.8	172
Cottage cheese, whole milk	120	5.0	3.0	100
Cottage cheese, low-fat	100	2.5	1.5	100
Cottage cheese, non-fat	80	0	0	150

Calcium for Bones:
Dairy Alone Is Not Enough

Calcium is the most abundant mineral in the body, and most of it is stored in the bones and teeth. Dairy is a concentrated source of calcium, but it's not the only one. Others include green leafy vegetables, canned salmon and sardines with edible bones, and calcium-fortified products (such as orange juice and soy foods). Moreover, the key to strong bones and ultimately prevention of osteoporosis is not in how much calcium is consumed, but how much is actually absorbed and retained by the body.[12]

Calcium is a fussy little mineral, requiring the cooperation of other influences, including supportive minerals and dietary factors. Different nutrients are necessary to maintain enough calcium in the blood, thereby reducing the chances that the body will steal reserves from bones. Vitamin D, phosphorous, potassium, and magnesium are all important in maintaining the proper amount of calcium in blood and bones.

Some common components of a typical diet may make calcium absorption and sufficiency more difficult. For example:

✗ Excessive protein consumption appears to interfere with calcium uptake and may actually increase calcium loss.[13]

✗ Fiber binds to the mineral and blocks its absorption, so it may be best to eat super-high-fiber foods and high-calcium foods or supplements at different times.[14]

✗ Saturated fat also reduces the absorption of calcium[15]—another reason why low-fat and fat-free dairy products are a better choice.

✗ Caffeine can interfere with calcium absorption and also leech calcium from bones and increase its excretion in urine.[16] (See "About Caffeine," pages 229–231.)

All about Eggs

The USDA's Food Guide Pyramid groups eggs with meat, poultry, fish, beans, and nuts, but in the American Heart Association's Eating Plan, they're grouped separately and viewed as a fat. This should be example enough of the lost identity of the poor, beleaguered egg. But whatever their classification, one thing is true: ounce-per-ounce, eggs are one of most concentrated sources of nutrients, loaded with high-quality protein as well as vitamins A, D, and B_{12}, and iron. Eaten in moderation (up to 3 or 4 eggs a week), they can be a part of a healthy diet.

Shopping Tips: Making the Grade

Eggs get higher grades depending on quality and appearance of the egg and its shell.

Grade AA eggs have firm, stand-up yolks, with a smaller white area and more thick white than thin white. Use them for poached eggs or for dishes in which the appearance of the egg is important. After ten days, Grade AA eggs become Grade A.

Grade A eggs are slightly less firm, but still have a thick white. They're best used for frying and in other recipes requiring eggs.

Grade B eggs have a slightly thinner white and flatter yolk. They're best used for scrambling or in cooking.

What about brown eggs? They may seem more nutritious, due to culture cues, but they're no different from white, just from different breeds of hens.

For those concerned about the conditions in which egg-laying chickens are caged—crowding, sanitation issues, use of antiobiotics, and other factors—eggs produced in alternative ways are available. For example:

Free-range eggs come from hens that have more movement, fresh air, and sunlight.

Fertile eggs have the same nutritional lineup as non-fertile eggs, but the hens have been allowed more freedom of movement, including consorting with roosters.

Organic eggs come from hens that have not been given drugs or antibiotics and are fed on organic grains.

Not So Heartbreaking After All?

The cholesterol in eggs has given them a bad rap, despite the powerful nutrient punch they pack. It is common knowledge that high blood cholesterol levels correlate with high risk for cardiovascular disease. Yet for most people, dietary cholesterol is less of a culprit than saturated fat in raising blood cholesterol levels.[17, 18] And since the fat in eggs is primarily monounsaturated, over-easy may be less heartbreaking than is traditionally thought.

Even so, it is hard to tell if any individual is sensitive to cholesterol consumption. (The study just cited showed a higher incidence of heart attacks and strokes among people with diabetes who averaged one egg daily.) The bottom line: moderation is still key.

A recent study from the Harvard School of Public Health showed that healthy people who ate up to 7 eggs per week did not increase their risk of heart attack or stroke.[19]

Incidentally, cholesterol-free and reduced-cholesterol egg substitutes are available. The taste is a poor substitute for whole eggs. Using the white from whole eggs, with a little turmeric added for yellow color, serves the same purpose without sacrificing taste, and without the artificial ingredients and flavors usually included in egg substitutes.

Storage and Safety

The potential for food poisoning from eggs raises safety issues when storing and eating eggs.

Salmonella bacteria is the main culprit in egg-related food poisoning. It was originally thought that if the shells were cleaned and the eggs were not cracked, the salmonella bacteria were not a problem. It is now known that salmonella can spread from an infected hen into the eggs, so extra caution is required. Some safe handling tips:

✗ Keep raw and cooked eggs refrigerated at temperatures of less than 40° F.

✗ Do not get egg shells wet. Water makes the shell more porous and can introduce infection.

✗ Never eat raw eggs in any form. This includes eggnog and Caesar salad dressing made with raw eggs. Avoid soft-cooked and undercooked eggs as well. Eggs should be cooked for a minimum of 3 minutes.

✗ After cooking eggs, serve or refrigerate immediately.

✗ Use leftover cooked eggs within 4 days.

✗ Never eat eggs that have been out of the refrigerator for more than 2 hours. Be careful with egg dishes at picnics and in brown bag lunches.

Meat & Poultry...

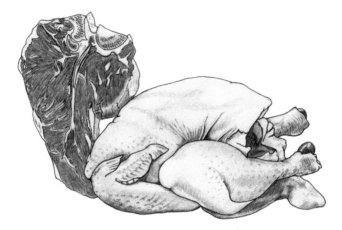

Meat has long been the defining factor in cultural traditions and celebrations, from the ceremonial slaughtering of pigs in ancient Greece to the grilling of burgers on the Fourth of July. Meat and poultry can have an important place in a satisfying, balanced, and healthy diet. The key is moderation.

Meat is a source of complete protein and contains vitamin B_{12}, the only vitamin that is difficult to get in a vegetarian diet. It also has high levels of zinc, iron, and other B vitamins. On the downside, meat and poultry can be high in saturated fat and cholesterol (to varying degrees) and have no fiber.

How Much Is Enough?

The American Heart Association recommends no more than 6 ounces of cooked lean meat, skinless poultry, or fish per day.[1] A serving is equivalent to 3 ounces of cooked (4 ounces raw) meat or poultry, about the size of a deck of playing cards. Some examples:

✗ a small hamburger
✗ ¼ of a chicken breast
✗ ½ cup of ground turkey
✗ 3 ounces of pork loin
✗ 2 thin slices of roast beef

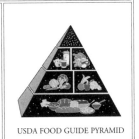

USDA FOOD GUIDE PYRAMID

Shopping Tips

When selecting meat, choose poultry and lower-fat cuts. Examples include chicken breast, turkey breast, lean beef (round, sirloin, chuck, loin) in "choice" or "select" grades, lean or extra-lean (less than 15 percent fat) ground beef, lean ham and pork, lean lamb (leg, arm, and loin cuts), and wild game. Higher-fat (and preferably avoided) meats include "prime" grade cuts and domesticated game birds, such as duck and goose.

Hygiene and Storage

Handle meat carefully to prevent the spread of harmful bacteria like E. coli and salmonella. Make sure meat is cold when it's purchased, and place the unopened package of meat in a plastic bag to prevent blood and juices from dripping onto other foods. Keep raw meat away from cooked food and produce. Thoroughly wash with a disinfectant all utensils and cutting boards used in meat preparation.

Store meat at temperatures of 38° F or less. Make sure to keep meat in the coldest portion of the freezer— all the way at the back. But don't forget about it—even frozen meat has a shelf life. A whole chicken or turkey will last about 12 months, a roast beef or steak 6 to 8 months, pork chops 3 to 6 months, ground beef 3 to 4 months, and a whole ham 1 to 2 months. Defrost meat in the refrigerator, never at room temperature.

Refrigerate leftover cooked meat immediately to prevent bacterial contamination, and separate large portions into smaller portions to speed cooling. Use cooked meat or poultry stored in the refrigerator within 3 to 4 days.

Whatever the cooking method, cook meat to an internal temperature of at least 180° F to destroy harmful bacteria. Rare isn't a safe option. Reheat leftovers by covering and heating to 165° F, or until hot and steaming throughout.

Meaty Issues

Unlike fruits and vegetables, which are hands-down winners in the healthy eating game, high consumption of meat is related to serious health concerns. The real beef is with the saturated fat in meat, which increases serum cholesterol levels and risk of cardiovascular disease and cancer.[2] For some people, the high cholesterol content in some meats can also be problematic.

✗ **Saturated fats** (fats that remain hard at room temperature) are found in animal foods like red meat, cheese, and butter, and in some vegetable products like coconut and palm oil. They're the main culprits in raising blood cholesterol and triglyceride levels.[3]

✗ **Cholesterol** is a soft, waxy steroid necessary in the formation of cell membranes and the production of hormones. Although the body needs cholesterol, the liver produces more than enough, so dietary sources are unnecessary.[4] Cholesterol is found only in animal foods, such as meat (especially organ meats), poultry, seafood, dairy products, and egg yolks. Shrimp and lobster are fairly high in cholesterol. Poultry and fish have about as much cholesterol as lean beef and pork. Dietary cholesterol is thought to be less of a factor in raising cholesterol levels than saturated fat; only about 10 percent of the population is sensitive to this effect.[5]

Research has consistently established a link between saturated fat intake and greater risk of disease, and a more tentative connection between meat consumption in particular and increased risk of certain kinds of cancer.[6]

As far back as 1990, the American Heart Association, American Cancer Society, National Academy of Sciences, American Academy of Pediatrics, and other advisory organizations were recommending that Americans reduce consumption of animal foods while reorienting toward a more vegetable-based diet.[7] Currently, the American Heart Association recommends that 30 percent or less of the day's total calories come from fat, with less than 10 percent of total calories from saturated fatty acids, and less than 300 mg of cholesterol.[8]

The total fat content varies widely among meats and poultry, from less than two grams in a 3-ounce serving of boneless, skinless chicken breast to the 26 grams in a serving of beef spareribs. Similarly, poultry breast is far lower in saturated fat than certain cuts of red meat, like beef ribs, pork ribs, and lamb chops.

In recent years, some cuts of pork have been promoted as "the other white meat"—in effect, as low-fat alternatives to chicken. Consider this comparison between 3-ounce servings of chicken breast (with skin) and pork tenderloin:

	Chicken breast	Pork tenderloin
Calories	170	150
Fat	7 grams	5 grams
Saturated fat	2 grams	2 grams
Cholesterol	70 mg	65 mg
Protein	25 grams	24 grams

Meat and Poultry[9]
(3-ounce serving; skin or visible fat not removed)

	Calories	Protein (grams)	Total fat (grams)	Saturated fat (grams)	Cholesterol (grams)
Chicken, breast	170	25	7	1.5	70
Chicken, thigh	210	22	13	4	80
Turkey, wing	200	23	11	3	70
Ground beef (27% fat)	250	15	17	6	85
Ground beef (10% fat)	210	15	11	4	85
Beef, brisket	290	10	21	8	80
Beef, sirloin steak	210	15	12	5	75
Beef top round, steak	180	15	7	3	85
Veal, chop	180	21	10	0	85
Veal, cutlet	140	24	4	0	85
Pork, ground	250	22	18	7	80
Pork, ham	155	15	9	3	48
Pork loin, roast	150	24	5	2	65
Lamb, chop	230	20	16	6	80
Lamb, leg	210	22	12	5	80

Preparation and Cooking: Cutting the Fat

A few simple steps while preparing and cooking meat can help limit fat consumption.

✘ Before cooking poultry in stews, soups, stir-fry dishes, and casseroles, remove the skin and the fat under the skin.

✘ Before cooking beef, pork, or lamb, trim off any visible fat on the surface.

Trimming the Fat[10]
(3-ounce serving)

	Calories	Fat (grams)	Saturated fat (grams)	Protein (grams)
Chicken breast				
—with skin	170	7	2	25
—without skin	120	1.5	0.5	24
Beef, chuck, pot roast				
—with fat	260	18	7	15
—visible fat trimmed	180	7	3	20
Pork, loin, sirloin roast,				
—with fat	220	14	5	23
—visible fat trimmed	180	9	3	25
Lamb, loin chop				
—with fat	250	18	7	22
—visible fat trimmed	180	8	3	25

✗ When roasting or broiling chicken or turkey, use a rack and drip pan to allow the fat to drip off. Then remove the skin after cooking.

✗ Chill soups and stews after cooking—the fat will rise to the surface and harden, making it easy to skim off.

Too Much Protein?

Most Americans are aware of the potential health hazards of consuming too much red meat and saturated fat. But what about lean meat and poultry? Independent of the fat factor, it's still not advisable to eat too much meat.

The problem is twofold. First, diets that focus on high-protein animal foods may tend to crowd out antioxidant and fiber-rich foods like fruits, vegetables,

To calculate your protein requirement... Convert your weight in pounds to kilograms by dividing by 2.2, then multiply by 0.8 grams. Thus, for someone weighing 160 pounds:

160 pounds ÷ 2.2 = 75 kg
75 x 0.8 = 60

This protein requirement of 60 grams per day is equivalent to the amount contained in 6 to 8 ounces of poultry or lean beef. Of course, protein is also available from other sources, such as dairy foods, legumes, nuts, and grains.

legumes, and grain products. Second, a high-protein diet can lead to nutrient imbalance and put a strain on the liver and kidneys.[11]

The World Health Organization recommends 10 to 15 percent of total calories from protein, or about 0.8 grams per kilogram of body weight.

Meat, Preservatives, and Drugs

In addition to saturated fat and cholesterol, other substances in some meats may pose health hazards. Consumption of preservatives added to smoked and cured meats may raise cancer risk, while antibiotics used in livestock production may increase the incidence of bacterial disease in humans. Improper inspection and handling of meat can lead to microbial contamination.

Preservatives. BHA, BHT, and propyl gallate are used to prevent discoloration and preserve freshness. Government-sponsored research has shown that BHT causes cancer in laboratory animals. Sodium nitrite, used as a preservative in luncheon meats, bacon, hot dogs and other processed meats, can combine with amino acids to form cancer-causing nitrosamines. The NIH's National Toxicology Program classes BHA, BHT, and sodium nitrite as likely human carcinogens.[12] It's a good idea to limit consumption of smoked and cured meats.

Antibiotics. Livestock producers routinely use antibiotics as a preventive measure, to control diseases that come from the strict confinement and crowded conditions on commercial ranches. Overuse of antibiotics in humans has contributed to a pool of resistant bacteria, and the use of subtherapeutic doses of antibiotics in livestock may contribute to this serious problem as well. A 1999 study, for instance, identified a significant increase in drug-resistant *Campylobacter jejuni* infections in humans due to the use of antibacterial agents (quinolones) in domestically-produced poultry.[13] According to a report published in 1999 by the National Research Council, "a link can be demonstrated between the use of antibiotics in food animals, the development of resistant microorganisms in those animals and the spread of pathogens to humans."[14]

Hormones. Drugs such as steroids and growth hormones are routinely administered to beef, lamb, and pork to promote weight gain and increase production.

Drug residues in animal-derived food products are an important consideration for consumers. Federal regulations allow for small quantities of drug residues in meat. Proponents of organic livestock-raising say even those tiny quantities may be unsafe in the long run. Allergenic, toxic, and carcinogenic effects are some of the possible long-term health consequences of consuming such residues in large quantities.[15] The European Economic Community banned hormone-treated meats in 1989, but they continue to be used in the United States.

Inhumane treatment of animals is another growing concern—and one that is being addressed by some livestock producers.

Organically-raised meats may be preferable for people interested in buying beef that is as untouched by commercial production processes as possible. They are available at natural food stores and larger supermarkets. Terms to look for include "organic," "free of antibiotics," "hormone free," "drug free," "humanely raised." (The term "natural" just means no additives were used in processing; it doesn't apply to production issues.)

License to grill?... Before heating up the barbecue, consider this: Cooking meat until it's very well done and has a blackened, crispy crust creates carcinogens called heterocyclic amines (HCAs). Women who regularly consume meat cooked to this degree over a very hot grill have been found to have nearly five times greater risk of breast cancer compared to women who prefer meat medium or rare.[16]

Frying meat to a well-done crisp can also generate HCAs. In one study, frying ground beef with 5 percent fat led to a five times higher concentration of HCAs than was created when frying meat with 15 percent fat. The extra fat may have an insulating effect, researchers say.[17]

To be prudent, grill only occasionally, and avoid grilling over very high heat. Covering the grill can keep the fire from flaming up. Partially pre-cooking foods in the microwave can shorten the time needed on the grill and help prevent blackened and crispy crusts. Limit consumption of fried meat.

Marinating meat in citrus juice or vinegar before grilling can reduce the formation of HCAs by 90 percent or more, according to the American Institute for Cancer Research.[18]

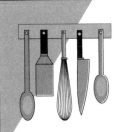

The center of the plate...
Given research findings that link heavy meat consumption with increased risk of disease, the key is to make a little meat go a long way. Take a hint from other cultures which use meat as a "condiment," with grains, beans, and vegetables making up the bulk of the main dish. Some examples:

✗ Toss cooked linguini or soba noodles with stir-fried snow peas, julienne sliced carrots, sliced water chestnuts, and a small amount of cooked chicken. Add a splash of soy sauce with a dash of ginger and some toasted sesame seeds for a fast Asian dinner dish.

✗ Make a Spanish-style paella: combine cooked rice, eggplant, potatoes, peppers, onions, mushrooms, and tiny bits of cooked lean ham or chicken. Season with ground cumin, black pepper, and garlic.

✗ Layer cooked black beans on warm, whole-wheat tortillas. Sprinkle with a little cooked, lean ground turkey and lots of chopped, very ripe tomatoes, Romaine lettuce, finely diced onions, and chopped cilantro for a light Mexican salad. Top with a small amount of grated low-fat cheese and a dollop of low-fat sour cream.

About Mad Cow Disease

In 1996, a new variant of Creutzfeldt-Jakob disease (vCJD)—a disease that causes lack of coordination, muscle twitching or jerking, dementia, and eventually, death— suddenly appeared in Great Britain. It is believed that the victims contracted the disease from eating the beef of cattle stricken with bovine spongiform encephalopathy (BSE). Otherwise known as "mad cow disease," BSE is a chronic neurodegenerative illness that has affected tens of thousands of cattle in Britain and 11 other countries. Cattle developed BSE after they were fed offal and other by-products from sheep carrying a neurodegenerative disease known as scrapie. As of December 1997, at least 25 people in the United Kingdom and France had contracted vCJD.[19, 20]

BSE has an incubation period of 3 to 8 years in cattle; CJD incubates in humans for about 13 years. According to the Federal Drug Administration, there are no reported cases of mad cow disease among cattle in the United States. Since 1985, no cattle has been imported from countries with native cattle cases of BSE, and no beef has been imported from any of these countries since 1989.[21] Nor has the Centers for Disease Control and Prevention detected any cases of vCJD in the U.S.[22] In June 1999, the American Medical Association's Council on Scientific Affairs reported that mad cow disease has not been shown to exist in this country, and that the "current risk of transmission of BSE in the United States is minimal."[23]

Fair Game

Venison, buffalo, rabbit, and other game meats are lower in fat, calories, and cholesterol than domesticated red meats. They're also free of hormones, antibiotics, additives, and preservatives. Use them instead of beef in sauces, stews, and burgers. To prevent drying, cook slowly over low heat.

Game Meats[24]
(3-ounce serving)

	Calories	Protein (grams)	Total fat (grams)	Saturated fat (grams)	Cholesterol (mg)
Buffalo	111	23	1.5	0.5	52
Rabbit	167	25	6.8	2.0	70
Venison	134	26	2.7	1.0	75
Ostrich	120	23	2.4	NA	72

Fish & Seafood...

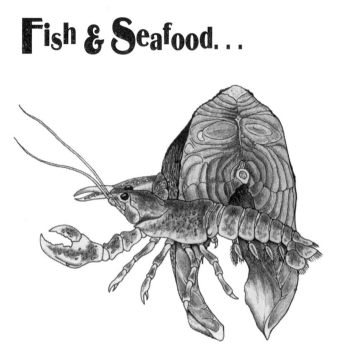

Since biblical times, fish and seafood have been a part of legend and lore, from sacred food to aphrodisiac. Fish continues to be the most widely consumed animal protein in the world—nearly 60 percent of the world's population looks to seafood to provide 40 percent of its animal protein. In Asian countries alone, about one billion people depend on seafood for *all* their animal protein. In 1997, Japanese ate nearly 33 pounds of fish per person. Americans consume about 14 pounds of fish per person every year.

Fish and seafood are excellent sources of protein, with much less fat and cholesterol than lean meat. They are good sources of minerals, including iron, zinc,

How Much Is Enough?

The American Heart Association recommends no more than 6 ounces of cooked lean meat, poultry, or fish per day. Yet the AHA has singled out fish as a "good source of protein without the accompanying high saturated fat seen in fatty meat products."[1] A serving size is equivalent to 3 ounces of cooked fish. Some examples:

✗ about half a salmon steak
✗ about half a small trout
✗ about ½ can of tuna
✗ a handful of steamed shrimp

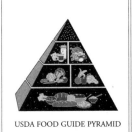

USDA FOOD GUIDE PYRAMID

magnesium, and phosphorous, and they also contain vitamins A and D. Because they contain less connective tissue than other flesh foods, fish and seafood are easier to digest than meat and poultry.

The most compelling reason to eat fish: it's loaded with omega-3 fatty acids, which can reduce susceptibility to cardiovascular and other disease.[2] Eating fish at least once a week has been linked to a lower risk of premature death.[3] (See "The Fatted Fish," page 125.)

Shopping Tips

Larger supermarkets are usually good sources for fish and seafood, since they have a higher demand and turnover. Avoid fish counters that look grimy. A reputable fish dealer will be well-informed about the various types of fish he or she sells, where and when they were caught, how long they've been on ice, and how they were processed or prepared.

When buying fish, it's prudent to smell it first. Fresh fish should not have a strong fishy odor—it should smell slightly sweet, like fresh seawater. All cuts of fish should be moist and firm, with a bright, almost translucent appearance. The color should be consistent. When shopping for whole fish, look for red gills, moist, firm, and bright skin, undamaged scales, and clear eyes. Avoid any fish with spotting, bruises, browning, or discoloration.

Pre-wrapped fish and seafood are harder to judge—more prudent to select from unwrapped options in the display case. If pre-wrapped is the only option, go ahead and purchase it, then open it before you leave the store. If it smells too fishy or feels slimy, return it immediately.

Sometimes fish is dipped in low-concentration chlorine to retard spoilage. This is probably safe, but people who don't want to consume chlorine might ask about this.

Frozen fish is another alternative. With advances in freezing technologies, the quality of frozen fish is greatly improved. If properly and immediately frozen, fish will retain its fresh flavor and texture, as well as nutrients.

Frozen fish should be solidly frozen and in tightly-wrapped packages free of ice buildup.

Be very careful with shellfish, since it's especially susceptible to bacterial contamination. Oysters, clams, mussels, crayfish, crab, and lobster should always be purchased live and, ideally, cooked immediately. Mollusks may be shucked and separated from their guts, which dramatically extends shelf life. Smell them first. Shrimp may be sold fresh or frozen, or frozen and thawed. They're safer when purchased still frozen.

Thawing. To be prudent, thaw frozen fish in the refrigerator. Placing it in a zip lock bag and then setting it in a bowl of cold water will speed thawing time. Thawing under cold running water is another option. To retain more moisture, don't thaw frozen fish completely before cooking. Cook and serve just like fresh fish.

Fish Varieties and Cooking Methods

The term "fish" refers to all fresh or saltwater finfish, mollusks and shellfish, crustaceans, and other forms of aquatic animal life. Dozens of varieties of fish are available in most supermarkets. Here are some basics.

White fish fillets are usually stark white, tender, and sweet, with a mild and delicate flavor, and are virtually fat-free. Catfish, dogfish, flounder, sole, dab, haddock, freshwater bass, freshwater pike, ocean perch, red snapper, rockfish, sea bass, and whiting fall apart easily and are best poached in a thick sauce or used in stews.

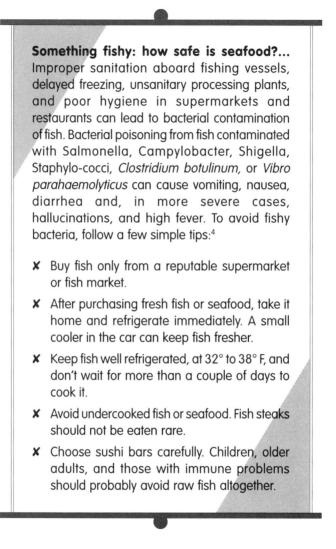

Something fishy: how safe is seafood?...
Improper sanitation aboard fishing vessels, delayed freezing, unsanitary processing plants, and poor hygiene in supermarkets and restaurants can lead to bacterial contamination of fish. Bacterial poisoning from fish contaminated with Salmonella, Campylobacter, Shigella, Staphylo-cocci, *Clostridium botulinum,* or *Vibro parahaemolyticus* can cause vomiting, nausea, diarrhea and, in more severe cases, hallucinations, and high fever. To avoid fishy bacteria, follow a few simple tips:[4]

✘ Buy fish only from a reputable supermarket or fish market.

✘ After purchasing fresh fish or seafood, take it home and refrigerate immediately. A small cooler in the car can keep fish fresher.

✘ Keep fish well refrigerated, at 32° to 38° F, and don't wait for more than a couple of days to cook it.

✘ Avoid undercooked fish or seafood. Fish steaks should not be eaten rare.

✘ Choose sushi bars carefully. Children, older adults, and those with immune problems should probably avoid raw fish altogether.

They may also be dredged in flour and sautéed. Since they cook very quickly (¼-inch-thick fillet may take as little as 3 minutes), they require some care in cooking. When the outside becomes opaque, the inside is almost

Fish and Seafood[5]
(3-ounce serving; cooked)

	Calories	Protein (grams)	Total fat (grams)	Saturated fat (grams)
Bluefish	135	22	4.6	1.0
Carp	137	19	6.1	1.2
Clams	126	22	1.7	0.2
Cod	89	19	0.7	0.1
Crab	86	17	1.5	0.2
Halibut	119	23	2.5	0.4
Herring	172	20	9.9	2.2
Lobster	83	17	0.5	0.1
Mackerel	222	20	15.1	3.5
Perch	99	21	1.0	0.2
Salmon	156	23	6.4	1.4
Salmon, canned	130	17	6.2	1.4
Salmon, smoked	99	16	3.7	0.8
Sardines, packed in oil	118	7	3.2	0.4
Sea bass	105	20	2.2	0.6
Shark	194	16	11.7	2.7
Shrimp	84	18	0.9	0.2
Snapper	108	22	1.5	0.3

Continued ➔

	Calories	Protein (grams)	Total fat (grams)	Saturated fat (grams)
Surimi	84	13	0.7	0.2
Swordfish	131	22	4.4	1.2
Trout	127	19	4.9	1.4
Tuna, fresh	156	25	5.3	1.4
Tuna, packed in oil	158	23	6.9	1.4
Tuna, packed in water	109	20	2.5	0.7
Tuna, light, in water	98	22	0.7	0.2
Whitefish, smoked	92	20	0.8	0.2
Whiting	99	20	1.4	0.3

done. For thicker fillets (up to 1 inch thick), 8 minutes is long enough.

Fish steaks are higher in omega-3s than white fillets, and have a slightly higher oil content. They're usually cut from larger ocean fish like swordfish, tuna, and salmon. On occasion, cod or whiting may be cut into steaks, but it is rare that they're permitted to grow large enough. Bluefish and mackerel are more delicate in texture but strong in flavor. Grouper, halibut, mahi mahi, mako, sturgeon, swordfish, tuna, and salmon lend themselves well to grilling, broiling, or poaching in broth or wine. Monkfish isn't a true steak but has a sturdy texture that allows it to be treated as one.

Fish tales... Literally speaking, there is no such thing as a sardine. Nor is there a fish called scrod. And Atlantic salmon isn't really salmon at all.

"Sardine," derived from the name of a Mediterranean island (Sardinia), refers to various kinds of small fish that have been processed and canned. Sardines from Scandinavia are usually brisling and silds. Those from Maine are small herrings, and those from France and Portugal are pilchards, a smaller, fatter variety of herring.

The name "scrod" comes from a Middle Dutch word "schrode" meaning a strip or shred. In New England, scrod are immature cod or haddock weighing 1½ to 2½ pounds.

Atlantic salmon is actually from the genus *Salmo,* or trout family. The misnomer is so widely accepted that it would only cause confusion to rename the species.

Salmon and trout are rich and oily, flavorful without tasting fishy. They're related in species and many farm-raised trout look and taste like salmon. Because of the high-fat content (rich in omega-3 fatty acids), they're fairly easy to cook. Salmon and trout can be poached, grilled, broiled, or pan cooked. If the fish is sold with the skin on, it may be scaled, skinned, or cooked with the skin. The latter is a good solution—just peel the skin off afterward and discard.

Dark fish fillets like bluefish and mackerel, as well as bonito, mullet, and pompano, are strong in flavor and, when cooked properly, rich and delicious. Dense and oily (rich in omega-3 fatty acids), they can be broiled, grilled, or simmered in sauce. They're especially good cooked with vinegar, tomato, or other tart ingredients that balance their strong flavor.

Shrimp are packed with protein and although relatively high in cholesterol, they're still lower in cholesterol than meats. Moreover, they may increase blood levels of HDL, or high-density lipoprotein, the "good" cholesterol.[6] Shrimp come in several varieties and sizes. Small, medium, and large are subjective categories, so it's best to judge them by the number it takes to make a pound. Shrimp labeled "16–20," for example, means there are 16 to 20 shrimp in a pound. In those labeled "U20," less than 20 make a pound. Shrimp in the range of 15 to 30 per pound usually have the best flavor and value. Shrimp may be peeled and cooked in sauces, sautéed in olive oil, grilled or stir-fried, or cooked with the shell on and then peeled before eating.

The black stripe or "vein" under the shrimp's skin is actually the shrimp's intestinal tract. Deveining (before or after cooking) is optional.

Crab and lobster have sweet, white meat that's low in fat and high in protein. They're best purchased live, or they may be purchased cooked and frozen or refrigerated. Lobster and crabs should be lively—pick them up before purchasing them. If they're not moving much, they're not fresh. The easiest cooking methods are boiling or steaming. Serve them either hot or cold.

Mollusks include clams, mussels, scallops, and oysters. Since they spoil rapidly, they should always be purchased fresh. Scallops may be the exception to this rule: because their shells never close completely, they're shucked right after harvest and gutted to prevent spoilage. Mollusks can be steamed or boiled in their shells, baked with stuffing, or shucked and cooked in stews, sauces, or stir-fry dishes.

A Good Catch: Alternatives to Fresh Fish

For those not up to the task of buying, storing, or preparing fresh or frozen fish, smoked and canned fish can boost omega-3 fatty acid levels and add a fast source of low-fat protein to any meal plan.

Frozen fish dinners. Depending on how they're prepared, frozen fish dinners can be a healthier alternative to meat. Just avoid breaded fillets, fish sticks, and entrées with artificial preservatives, oils, and excess salt.

Smoked fish. Smoked fish was traditionally cured with smoke and salt to preserve it. Modern smoked fish is cured using a different process, the goal being flavor rather than preservation. To serve smoked fish, arrange slivers on salads, or serve on crackers or bagels with sliced tomatoes, finely minced onions, and capers.

The fatted fish... Omega-3s are the good-for-you polyunsaturated fatty acids that make fish so healthy. Essential for the normal functional development of the retina and brain,[7] they are abundant in fattier fish like salmon, sardines, mackerel, tuna, and herring, and present in smaller amounts in white fish and other seafoods. Studies have shown that, among other important health benefits, omega-3s:

✗ lower blood cholesterol and triglyceride levels and reduce blood pressure[8]

✗ decrease the risk of heart disease[9]

✗ help protect against sudden cardiac death[10]

✗ ease the symptoms of rheumatoid arthritis and other inflammatory conditions[11]

Omega-3 Sources
(3½-ounce serving)

Sardines, packed in water	3.0 grams
Mackerel	2.5 grams
Salmon, pink	2.2 grams
Tuna	2.1 grams
Shark	1.9 grams
Herring	1.6 grams
Salmon, Atlantic	1.4 grams
Sablefish	1.3 grams
Rainbow trout	1.1 grams

(See also "Essential Knowledge: The ABCs of EFAs," pages 165–166.)

Sodium nitrites, which may be added to smoked fish, are used to inhibit the growth of the bacterium (*Clostridium botulinum*) that causes botulism. Yet according to the Federal Drug Administration's Center for Food Safety, regular consumption of nitrites may pose some cancer risk.[12] Those who are uncomfortable with this potential danger may choose nitrite-free varieties of smoked fish. Another option is to consume vitamin C (such as in citrus juice) along with smoked fish. Vitamin C inhibits the formation of nitrosamines, the carcinogens formed in the body from nitrites.[13]

Canned fish. Canned fish packed in water is a convenient, healthy way to add protein and omega-3s to the diet, with only 1 gram of fat per 4-ounce serving. Look for canned salmon and canned (water-packed) tuna. Chunk light tuna may include two or more species of tuna. Solid white tuna is from Albacore, and can be used in casseroles and stir-fry dishes instead of chicken breast. For those who want to try something different with canned tuna, how about stir-frying it with diced vegetables, a splash of low-sodium soy sauce, and a spoonful of sesame seeds. Mix canned salmon with fat-free yogurt, fresh dill and black pepper, and serve on dark bread.

Sardines. Loaded with omega-3 fatty acids, sardines are also a good source of fast protein. They may be packed in oil, brine, or a variety of savory sauces. The brine-packed or sauce-packed varieties have less fat. Serve them the traditional European way: broiled for about 10 minutes and served with lemon wedges, minced parsley, and hot sourdough bread.

Surimi. Surimi is a processed fish product most often encountered in Japanese restaurants and sushi bars, where it's used instead of crab. Also known as "fake crab legs," it is usually made from pollock. The healthy fish oils are removed and the product is bleached to create a colorless, tasteless paste. The paste is then formed to look like various kinds of shellfish, and is loaded with artificial flavors and colors. It contains ample protein, but none of the healthy fish fats. Not a great substitute for fish.

Troubled Waters

As our modern world continues to develop, our water sources are becoming more and more endangered. Industrial and agricultural chemicals and other sources of toxins including raw sewage, runoff, improperly stored wastes, and residues from abandoned dumps wash into lakes, streams, and coastal waters, where they concentrate in the fatty tissues of fish.

One contaminant, mercury, has been linked to nervous system damage. Mercury becomes tightly bound to proteins in fish tissue, so no method of cooking or cleaning fish will reduce the amount of mercury. PCBs, another contaminant that concentrates in the fatty tissues of fish, are synthetic oils linked to infant development problems and cancer. Although banned in 1976, PCBs remain in the water and sediment for many years. PCBs in fish cannot be fully removed through cleaning and cooking.[14]

Some tips for protecting yourself from toxins in fish:

✗ Choose wild ocean fish harvested hundreds of miles offshore.

✗ Choose farm-raised freshwater fish (trout, catfish, etc.).

✗ Buy fresh salmon caught during the Alaskan salmon season, early May to early September. Off-season, frozen Alaskan salmon is a better bet.

✗ Eat a variety of fish to reduce the risk of overdoing it on one toxic source.

✗ Limit fish consumption to two or three times a week. (Pregnant women shouldn't eat more than 7 ounces of canned tuna per week or fish from inland waters more than once a month.)

✗ Don't eat the skin of fish since it's a main storage area for toxins.

Legumes...

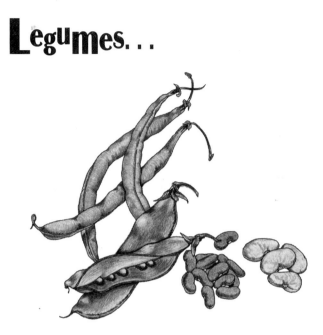

These versatile, savory staples—including beans, lentils, peas, and peanuts—are among the most widely consumed foods in the world. The ubiquitous bean, for example, plays a part in meals in every culture, showing up in soups, salads, side dishes, and sometimes in desserts. Until the advent of soy-mania, beans had a bad rap: they were thought to be fattening, hard to cook, and impossible to digest. If you believe these rumors, you don't know beans about legumes.

Legumes are high in folate, B vitamins, vitamin E, and the minerals calcium, magnesium, potassium, phosphorous, chlorine, sulfur, and iron. They contain 14 to 18 grams of protein per cup—more than any other plant food—and are extremely low in fat, with less than

How Much Is Enough?

Dry beans, peas, and lentils can be counted as servings in either the meat and beans group or the vegetable group. Three to five servings of vegetables are recommended. A serving of beans is equivalent to about ½ cup of cooked dried beans. Some examples:

✗ a handful of garbanzo beans on a salad
✗ a cup of lentil soup
✗ 4 ounces of canned peas
✗ ½ cup of tofu
✗ a small bean burrito

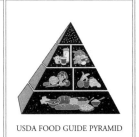

USDA FOOD GUIDE PYRAMID

1 gram of fat per cup and no saturated fat or cholesterol. A ½-cup serving of beans fulfills over 25 percent of the daily recommendation for fiber; the soluble fiber abundant in legumes can help lower serum cholesterol and stabilize blood sugar.[1, 2, 3] Half-a-cup of beans supplies over 50 percent of the recommended intake of folate, which, like fiber, is associated with reduced risk for cardiovascular illness.[4] Legumes also contain compounds believed to protect against cancer.[5,6] Considering their high protein and fiber content and their phytochemical punch, legumes are an excellent food smart choice, and a very economical one as well.

Shopping and Storage Tips

Most supermarkets carry a colorful selection of beans in every possible form. Look for dried beans prepackaged, or in the bulk section of some markets. Beans should be whole, smooth, and bright (dull and wrinkled beans with cracked seams are older and less flavorful). Store them in glass jars in a cool, dark location. Dried beans and legumes will keep for up to two years, but for maximum flavor and nutrition, use them within six months.

Canned beans are a quick and easy alternative, with not much lost in the way of nutrients. When using canned beans, don't discard the liquid—it contains some soluble fiber, minerals, and thiamin. Buy low-sodium varieties to avoid excess salt.

Beans[7]
(½-cup serving)

	Calories	Fiber (grams)	Folate (mcg)	Sodium (mg)
Pinto, boiled	117	7.4	147	2
Pinto, canned	103	5.5	72	353
Kidney, boiled	112	6.5	115	2
Kidney, canned	109	8.2	65	436
Garbanzo, boiled	135	6.2	141	6
Garbanzo, canned	143	5.3	80	359
Black, boiled	114	7.5	128	1
Black, canned	109	8.3	73	460

Cooking Legumes

Beans are one of the easiest foods to prepare. Just put them in a pot, add water, and boil. (For tips on soaking beans before cooking, see "Hold the Gas, Please," pages 134–135.) Most legumes take a couple of hours to cook, but using a pressure cooker shortens the time considerably. Lentils and split peas cook in only half an hour, without the pressure cooker.

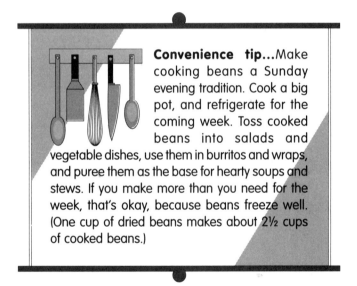

Convenience tip... Make cooking beans a Sunday evening tradition. Cook a big pot, and refrigerate for the coming week. Toss cooked beans into salads and vegetable dishes, use them in burritos and wraps, and puree them as the base for hearty soups and stews. If you make more than you need for the week, that's okay, because beans freeze well. (One cup of dried beans makes about 2½ cups of cooked beans.)

Bean around the World

All cooking times indicated below are for soaked beans.

Azuki (or **adzuki**). These small, dark red beans are native to Asia and commonly used as a traditional remedy for kidney ailments. Cooking time: 1½ hours.

Anasazi. Similar to pinto beans, these burgundy and white speckled beans were originally grown by Native Americans. Cooking time: 1½ hours.

Black beans. Small, compact black beans are especially popular in Mexican and Southwestern cooking. Cooking time: 1½ hours.

Black-eyed peas. Sometimes called cow peas, black-eyed peas are a staple in Southern kitchens. Cooking time: 1 hour.

Garbanzo. Also known as chickpeas, garbanzos are a staple food in Middle Eastern, Indian, and Mediterranean cuisine. Cooking time: 3 hours.

Kidney beans. Red beans named for their distinctive shape, kidney beans are traditionally used in Mexican and Southwestern meals. Cooking time: 1½ hours.

Lentils. These small, disk-shaped legumes, members of the pea family, range in color from brown to orange, red, and green. French lentils are smaller, with a dark grayish-blue color. Cooking time: 20 to 40 minutes.

Lima beans. Also called butter beans, lima beans have a rich, buttery flavor, and are traditionally used in Southern cooking and in traditional American succotash. Cooking time: 1½ hours.

Mung beans. Tiny, round, and green, mung beans are used primarily in Indian and African cooking. Sprouted mung beans are used in Asian cooking and stir-fry dishes. Cooking time: 1¼ hours.

Navy beans. These hefty white beans are traditionally used in Russian cooking and in hearty stews. Cooking time: 2½ hours.

Split peas. Flavorful, fast-cooking, and yellow or green, split peas belong to the legume family and are a mainstay of hearty soups. Cooking time: 45 minutes.

Pinto beans. These medium-sized beans are used mostly in Southwestern and Mexican cooking. Cooking time: 2 hours.

Soybeans. A staple food in Asia for thousands of years, the soybean, in its various incarnations, from tofu to tempeh to soy dairy substitutes, is now one of America's favorite legumes. Cooking time: 3 to 4 hours.

Hold the Gas, Please: Cooking Bloat-Free Beans

Beans contain complex sugars called oligosaccharides, which, among other effects, can lower blood sugar in people with diabetes. They are added to Glucerna® and other products for this purpose. But the not-so-good news about oligosaccharides is that they make beans hard for many people to digest. Oligosaccharides pass undigested into the lower intestine and are fermented by bacteria, thus producing gas.

Some beans—lentils, mung beans, and adzuki beans—tend to be easier to digest. Navy, lima, and soybeans are the toughest. Fortunately, certain preparation techniques can maximize digestibility and nutritional value.

✗ First, pick out stones and debris.

✗ Soak the beans before cooking (with the exception of lentils, mung beans, and split peas). The short soak method is best: boil beans for 5 minutes, cover and set aside for 2 or 3 hours, then drain and rinse thoroughly. Or cover them in water and let soak for 8 hours or overnight. The foam that rises to the top while beans soak is a sign that the complex carbohydrates are being broken down (that's what they would normally do in your gut).

✗ After soaking, place beans in a large pot and add 4 cups of water for each cup of dry beans. Be sure to use a tight cover.

✗ Adding a 4-inch strip of kombu sea vegetable speeds cooking time, makes beans more digestible (due to the glutamic acid content, which breaks down indigestible sugars), and adds flavor and valuable minerals. It is available at natural food stores and Japanese food markets. Cumin and bay leaf also assist with digestion and enhance flavor. (Don't use salt during cooking—it makes beans tough.)

✗ Cook thoroughly. For maximum digestibility and minimum gas, beans should be soft, not just tender.

If you're not used to eating lots of beans, make sure to start with small portions, giving your body time to adjust.

Oh, Boy—More on Soy

The wunderkind of the health foods scene, soy can help prevent cancer, lower cholesterol, ward off osteoporosis, and lessen the effects of menopause.[8, 9] Tofu, miso, tempeh, and soy-based dairy substitutes are among the numerous soy foods available. Most of the health benefits of soy have been attributed to its high concentration of phytoestrogens, including genistein and other isoflavones, which resemble natural estrogens in the body. Some highlights:

✘ Genistein in soy can lower risk for breast, colon, and prostate cancer.[10, 11]

✘ Soy has been shown to reduce both overall cholesterol levels and LDL levels, (without affecting HDL levels), both critical in protecting against cardiovascular disease.[12]

✘ Soy isoflavones can help prevent osteoporosis. One of them, genistein, has been reported to be as active as estrogens in maintaining bone mass in animal studies.[13]

✘ Phytoestrogens in soy products can help alleviate the symptoms of menopause.[14] (Soy burgers are an exception. Most contain no phytoestrogens.)

It's hard to cast aspersions on the wonder-food of the '90s. But some researchers say soy is overrated, while others point to possible dangers if soy is consumed in large quantities. Specifically, studies have shown that soy may cause digestive problems which interfere with mineral absorption—the former due to trypsin inhibitors which block the functioning of certain pancreatic enzymes,[15] and the latter due to compounds called phytates in soy which bind to calcium, iron, zinc, and other minerals.[16] Human studies have tentatively linked excessive soy consumption to suppressed thyroid function, including hypothyroidism.[17] And animal studies suggest that the same compounds that ease or prevent menopausal symptoms may also adversely affect fertility[18] and could interfere with the hormonal and sexual development of children.[19] This has not been shown in humans, however.

These findings await confirmation from further research. But they are worth considering, especially among those who might overdo it with soy. On the other hand, soy foods have long been consumed in abundance in Asia, without reported problems.

The potential detrimental effects of too much soy apparently do not apply to fermented soy foods like miso, tempeh, and natto—since fermentation prompts chemical changes that make soy more digestible and deactivate potentially harmful substances.

Nuts & Seeds...

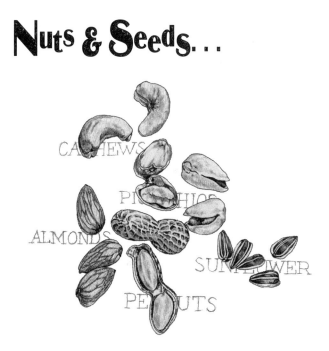

CASHEWS

PISTACHIOS

ALMONDS

SUNFLOWER

PEANUTS

Healthy or not? Nuts and seeds are a source of some confusion. As the nutritional storage unit of plants, they're highly-concentrated (read: high in calories) sources of the essential ingredients needed to produce a mature plant. But in moderation, they can be a healthy addition to any diet.

Nuts and seeds are good sources of protein, vitamin E, and B vitamins like folate, minerals, and phytochemicals that help protect against cancer and heart disease. They're also high in essential fatty acids (EFAs), which protect cardiovascular health. And the fats in nuts and seeds are of the heart-healthy, polyunsaturated and monounsaturated varieties.

How Much Is Enough?

Because of their fat content, nuts and seeds should be used sparingly. The American Heart Association classifies them with fats and oils, while the USDA Food Guide Pyramid includes them in the meat group. One-third cup of nuts or 2 tablespoons of peanut butter, for example, counts as 1 ounce of meat.

Shopping and Storage Tips

Raw and dry-roasted nuts and seeds have similar nutrient profiles, although there is some loss of nutrients in the roasting process. Unsalted versions are preferable, for obvious reasons. Buy whole nuts instead of chopped or sliced. Once a nut is cut or broken, its oils are exposed to air and oxidation occurs, producing potentially-harmful free radicals. Make sure they're fresh—old nuts and seeds have dark spots and taste sharp or bitter, a sign that the oils have gone rancid.

Nut and seed butters are a convenient way to add healthy fats to any diet, as a more nutritious alternative to butter. For those who would prefer to avoid the added salt, sugar, and other unnecessary ingredients in most commercial peanut butters, alternatives include organic and 100 percent nut and seed butters, without added salt or sugar. (See "Nut and Seed Butters," page 205.)

Stored in the refrigerator, most nuts and seeds will keep for up to six months. Refrigerate nut butters to prevent the oils from going rancid.

Nuts[1]
(1-ounce serving)

	Calories	Fat (grams)	Vitamin E* (I.U.)	Folate (mcg)	Sodium (mg)
Peanuts, raw	161	14	3.9	68	5.1
Peanuts, dry-roasted, salt added	166	14	3.2	41	230
Peanuts, dry-roasted, without salt	166	14	3.2	41	15
Almonds, dried unblanched	167	15	10.2	17	3.1
Almonds, dried blanched	167	15	8.6	11	2.8
Almonds, dry-roasted, unsalted	166	15	2.3	18	3.1
Almonds, dry-roasted, salt added	166	15	2.3	18	221
Cashews, dry-roasted, unsalted	163	13	0.3	20	4.5
Cashews, dry-roasted, salt added	163	13	0.3	20	181
Soy nuts, dry-roasted, unsalted	90	2	0.8	0	2.5

*Recommended intake of vitamin E is 10 I.U. (International Units) for men, 15 I.U. for women.

Go Nuts!

The key to healthy nut and seed use is the kind and quantity consumed. Tempting as it may be, it's not a good idea to eat salted, honey-roasted peanuts by the handful—before you know it, you'll have put away hundreds of calories and thousands of milligrams of salt. Instead, add small quantities of chopped nuts and seeds to fruits, vegetables, beans, and grains. Sprinkle ground flaxseed over fresh steamed vegetables. Add chopped walnuts to rice and bean dishes. Toss slivers of almonds into fruit salads for a nutty taste and a dose of healthy fats.

Here's a rundown of some of the many varieties of nuts and seeds.

Almonds. Grown primarily in California and Spain, the almond is the kernel of a small tree fruit, closely related to plums, peaches, and apricots. The highest source of calcium of all nuts as well as rich in heart-healthy vitamin E, almonds help lower cholesterol. (See "Health Nuts," page 145.)

Brazil nuts. Technically not a nut but a fruit, Brazil nuts grow wild in the Amazon Valley, and are the only commercial nuts that are still foraged. Brazil nuts are high in selenium, an essential trace mineral and antioxidant.

Cashews. From the fruit of the cashew evergreen tree, cashews are grown primarily in India and Brazil. They have the lowest fat of any nut besides the chestnut.

Chestnuts. Usually imported from Europe (ever since a blight early in this century wiped out nearly all of our native chestnuts), chestnuts have a light, sweet flavor and the lowest fat content of any nut.

Flaxseed. From the same plant used to produce linen and certain kinds of paint, flaxseeds are rich in essential fatty acids. They have become a popular complementary treatment for cardiovascular problems.

Facts about flax... What's the big deal about flax? Cultivated in Babylon as early as 3,000 BC, flax was considered so valuable in 8th century Rome that laws strictly governed its consumption. Also known as linseed, flax is the basis for linen fabric and certain kinds of paint. But current enthusiasm about flax focuses on the nutrient punch these little seeds pack, including *lignins* and *alpha-linolenic acids*—compounds thought to prevent disease.

Lignins are converted in the digestive tract into phytoestrogens that may block the growth of hormone-related cancers, like breast and colon cancer.[2] Flax is one of the best food sources of lignins: ¼ cup has as much lignin as five loaves of whole-wheat bread. Meanwhile, alpha-linolenic essential fatty acid is converted in the body to omega-3 fatty acid, which helps prevent heart disease, arthritis, and symptoms of menopause.[3, 4] (See "Essential Knowledge: The ABCs of EFAs," page 165–166.)

Hazelnuts. A member of the birch family, hazelnuts (also called filberts) get about 90 percent of their calories from fat, but most of it is the healthy variety. They are also one of the richest food sources of vitamin E.

Macadamia nuts. Commercially grown primarily in Hawaii and California, macadamia nuts have the highest percentage of calories from fat (95 percent), but most of it is healthy monounsaturated fat.

Peanuts. Cultivated by the ancient Aztecs and now grown in the southern United States, peanuts are technically a legume (they're sometimes called "ground nuts"), and they are among the lower-fat nuts.

Pecans. Pecans are cultivated mainly in the Mississippi River basin and other areas of the Southeastern United States. They're about 87 percent fat, mostly monounsaturated.

Pine nuts. Also called pignolia or piñon, the pine nut comes from the Piñon tree, grown primarily in Mexico, New Mexico, and the Mediterranean. Pine nuts are higher in protein than other nuts.

Pistachios. Known for its lovely green color, the pistachio is cultivated mainly in Turkey, Iran, and Afghanistan. It has the highest iron and potassium content of any nut.

Poppy seeds. Used primarily for appearance in cooking, poppy seed is believed to have calming effects and has been used as a traditional herbal remedy. Incidentally, in moderate quantities, poppy seed can cause a positive result on some drug tests.

Health nuts... Regular consumption of nuts can decrease one's chances of dying from heart-related causes, according to the American Heart Association and the results from a study of more than 22,000 male doctors.[5] Nuts are high in unsaturated fatty acids and magnesium, which may help prevent heart-rhythm disturbances, while their vitamin E content may limit the oxidation of lipids that contributes to atherosclerotic and other degenerative changes. Other nutty highlights:

✗ **Walnuts** decrease total serum levels of total cholesterol, lower LDL (the "bad cholesterol"), and increase HDL cholesterol levels.[6]

✗ **Brazil nuts** can prevent certain kinds of cancer, possibly by virtue of their high selenium content.[7]

✗ **Almonds** can help lower total cholesterol, decreasing LDL levels while preserving HDL levels.[8, 9]

✗ **Pumpkin seeds** may help treat symptomatic benign prostatic hyperplasia (BPH) in men (Stage I or II).[10]

Pumpkin seeds. From a special variety of pumpkin grown in Mexico, pumpkin seeds are also called "pepitas." They are thought to dispel intestinal parasites, and may help relieve symptoms of benign prostatic hyperplasia (BPH).

Sesame seeds. Traditionally used in Middle Eastern and Asian cooking, sesame seeds were once prized for their magical properties. Black sesame seeds are stronger in flavor and add interest to Japanese dishes. Both varieties are high in protein.

Soy nuts. Not really nuts at all, "soy nuts" have about one-half the calories of most nuts and are high in fiber (3 grams per ¼ cup), in addition to the healing phytochemicals in other soy foods.

Sunflower seeds. Indigenous to the United States, sunflower seeds are collected from the dried heads of sunflowers. They are high in protein and folate.

Walnuts. Originating in Persia, and used extensively in Russian and Middle Eastern cooking, walnuts now come mainly from California. They're high in omega-3 fatty acids and can help decrease cholesterol levels.

Grow Your Own

Sprouts are a great source of energy that add crunch and concentrated nutrition to nearly any dish. Like soaking or cooking, sprouting also eases digestion of raw nuts and seeds, by deactivating the protease inhibitors they contain and facilitating the conversion of protein into animo acids and starches into simple sugars.[11]

Sprouting gives nuts and larger seeds a sweet, more legume-like flavor. Spicy radish sprouts, for example, work well on sandwiches instead of lettuce. Other options: add clover sprouts to salads, or toss a handful of sprouted sunflower seeds into soups and stir-fry dishes.

Sunflower Seeds[12]
(¼-cup serving)

	Calories	Protein (grams)	Fat (grams)	Vitamin E (I.U.)	Folate (mcg)	Sodium (mg)
Dried	205	8	17.5	27	82	1.1
With hull	66	3	5.5	7.7	26	0.4
Dry-roasted, no salt added	186	6	16	24	76	1.0
Dry-roasted, salt added	186	6	16	24	76	250

Any raw nut or seed can be sprouted. Alfalfa, clover, and radish seed are the most widely available. Store-bought sprouted seeds should be bright and healthy. Pass over any that are browning, dry, or slimy. Or grow your own, following a few simple steps.

✗ Place 1 tablespoon of alfalfa, clover, or radish seeds in a quart jar.

✗ Cover with filtered water and soak for about 6 hours.

✗ Drain the water, rinse in fresh water, and drain again.

✗ Cover the top of the jar with a piece of cheesecloth and secure it with a rubber band. Place the jar on its side.

✗ Rinse the seeds twice a day—just run cool water through the gauze, swirl the jar gently, pour the water out, and drain well.

✗ After about five days, your sprouts should be ready. During the last day of sprouting, place the jar in the sun for a few hours to let them become green with chlorophyll.

To sprout nuts (such as cashews or almonds), or pumpkin or sunflower seeds, place a handful of the whole nuts or seeds (broken or chopped ones won't work) in a quart jar, cover with filtered water, and soak for 8 to 10 hours. Then follow the rest of the instructions for sprouting seeds. Sprouting nuts is a shorter procedure. They're ready in two days, when a small nub appears at the end of the nut.

Vegetarian Alternatives...

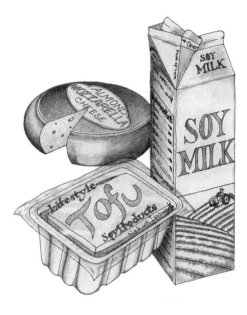

It used to be a statement, a quiet rebellion against the status quo, and a way to address issues such as the environment, world hunger, and economic and ethical considerations. In recent years, findings related to personal health have swelled the ranks of non-meat eaters, and there are now about 2 million vegetarians in the United States.[1]

Because of their lower saturated fat, zero cholesterol, and higher levels of phytochemicals, vegetarian diets have a protective effect against disease.[2] Compared to meat eaters, vegetarians have a lower rate of most chronic degenerative diseases[3, 4] and lower incidence of

Anything with a face?... Vegetarian used to mean one didn't eat anything that once walked, swam, flew—or to paraphrase the legendary Paul McCartney quote, anything with a face. In recent times, the lines have become more blurred. The most accepted divisions:

✗ **Vegan.** All animal products—including meat, fish, eggs, dairy, and honey—are avoided.

✗ **Lacto Vegetarian.** Milk, cheese, butter, and other dairy products are okay. Eggs and meat are avoided.

✗ **Ovo Vegetarian.** Eggs are okay, but meat, fish, and all dairy products are avoided.

✗ **Lacto-Ovo Vegetarian.** Dairy and eggs are eaten, but no flesh food, including fish.

✗ **Pesco Vegetarian.** Fish is okay. Other meat products, eggs, and dairy are avoided.

hypertension, independent of body weight and sodium intake.[5] They are less likely to die from Type II diabetes mellitus[6] and coronary artery disease[7] (while vegetarian diets low in saturated fat may actually help reverse severe coronary artery disease[8, 9]), and have a lower rate of lung and colorectal cancer.[10]

Vegetarian Eating and Nutrition

Would-be vegetarians worry about adequate intake of certain nutrients on a meat-free diet. With some attention to detail, vegetarians can get all the nutrients they need. Here are the facts about nutrients sometimes believed to be "missing" from vegetarian diets.

Protein. Non-meat sources of protein, like beans and dairy, can provide plenty of protein.[11] It was once thought that beans and grains had to be eaten at the same meal, to form a complete protein. (Vegetable proteins may be low in one or more essential amino acids, so mixing them ensures that the body has the necessary components to make complete proteins.) Now it's known that complementary proteins just need to be eaten on the same day.[12] Soy is the only plant food considered a complete protein.

Calcium. Meeting recommended calcium levels from food sources alone can be difficult for anyone, vegetarian or not. According to recent data, the average American consumes about 800 mg of calcium per day, with average consumption among women about 750 mg.[13] These are considerably short of recommended levels (1,000 to 1,200 mg per day for adults, 1,500 mg sometimes recommended for post-menopausal women).

Nonetheless, studies have shown that lacto-ovo vegetarians have calcium intakes comparable to or even higher than those of meat eaters.[14, 15] Vegans have lower calcium intakes, but they also have lower calcium needs, since diets lower in total protein have been shown to have a calcium-sparing effect.[16]

Calcium: Non-Dairy Sources[17]

	Amount	Calcium (mg)
Wakame	½ cup	1,700
Nori	½ cup	600
Kombu	¼ cup	500
Sesame seeds	¼ cup	500
Tempeh	1 cup	340
Turnip greens, cooked	1 cup	250
Collard greens, cooked	1 cup	240
Fortified rice milk	1 cup	280
Fortified soy milk	1 cup	280
Kale, cooked	1 cup	200
Mustard greens, cooked	1 cup	180
Broccoli	1 cup	178
Almonds	¼ cup	175
Tofu	1 cup	150
Navy beans	1 cup	140
Soybeans	1 cup	130
Pinto beans	1 cup	100
Walnuts	¼ cup	70
Sunflower seeds	¼ cup	70

Moreover, plant sources can provide ample calcium. For instance, 1 serving of tofu or a cup of most greens has nearly as much calcium as a glass of milk. Sesame seeds, broccoli, and sea vegetables are good sources of calcium, and many vegetarian foods like orange juice and soy milk are now calcium-fortified. Another plus is that calcium is absorbed efficiently from plant sources.[18]

Iron. Studies have shown that vegetarians do not have higher rates of iron-deficiency anemia than those of the general population.[19] The higher vitamin C content of vegetarian diets may even improve iron absorption.[20] And legumes and dark green vegetables have more iron per calorie than most meats.

Vitamin B_{12}. The requirements for vitamin B_{12} are small, and B_{12} is stored and recycled in the body for years.[21] Dairy products and eggs contain vitamin B_{12}, and many vegan foods are fortified with vitamin B_{12}. One word of caution: some of the vitamin B_{12} in tempeh, miso, spirulina, and sea vegetables is inactive B_{12} analog, rather than the active vitamin. Strict vegans should look for fortified soy milk and meat substitutes, and take a vegetarian B_{12} supplement.[22]

Vitamin D. Although vegan diets may be deficient in vitamin D, since fortified milk is the most prevalent dietary source, studies suggest that dietary intake of vitamin D is only important in the absence of sun exposure.[23] As little as 5 to 15 minutes of sun exposure per day should provide plenty of vitamin D,[24] although this may be a problem in cold climates, particularly in winter. Many vegetarian foods, like bread and soy milk, are fortified with vitamin D.

Essential fatty acids. Diets that don't include fish or eggs lack omega-3 fatty acids, and some vegetarians may have lower blood lipid levels of this fatty acid, though findings are contradictory.[25, 26] Flaxseed and walnuts, as well as canola oil and soybean oil, are good vegetarian sources of omega-3 fatty acids.

Zinc. Meat, eggs, and dairy foods are the most common dietary sources of zinc, but studies have generally found normal zinc levels even among vegans.[27] Soybeans and other legumes, sesame seeds, nuts, whole grains, and wheat germ are good vegetarian sources of zinc. RDAs for zinc are:[28]

✗ 10 mg for ages 1 to 10
✗ 15 mg for males ages 11+
✗ 12 mg for females ages 11+
✗ 15–19 mg during pregnancy and lactation

Plant Sources of Zinc

Food	Zinc (mg)
Wheat germ (¼ cup)	4.5
Wheat bran (½ cup)	3.5
Pumpkin seeds (1 ounce)	3.0
Sesame seeds (1 ounce)	2.0
Tofu (½ cup)	2.0
Sunflower seeds (1 ounce)	1.5
Almonds (1 ounce)	1.0
Peanut butter (1 ounce)	1.0

Phony Baloney:
The Best Meat Alternatives

Gooey tofu isn't the only choice for today's vegetarians. Here's a roundup of the meatiest solutions. One note: supermarket meat substitutes are often high in sodium and additives. It's worth a trip to the health food store for cleaner alternatives.

Tofu. Firm tofu holds its shape well and works best in stir-fries and soups. Silken tofu is soft and creamy, and is better for blended salad dressings and sauces. Baked tofu comes in a variety of flavors and makes a great high-protein snack on the go. Stick with the low-fat varieties for the most health benefits. Low-fat tofu has about 90 calories and 10 grams of protein per serving.

Nothing's perfect, not even tofu. Some researchers say soy is overrated, and may even cause health problems in large quantities. The best advice: vary tofu with other soy products (like tempeh and miso) and eat a variety of beans, not just soy, for high-fiber, low-fat sources of protein. (See "Oh, Boy—More on Soy," pages 136–137.)

Tempeh. This fermented soybean product has a distinctive taste and is much firmer than tofu. Slice it for stir-fries, crumble it in soups, or cube it for baking. It can also be marinated for extra flavor. Tempeh comes in a wide range of varieties, and may contain grains, vegetables, and seaweeds. Most versions have about 120 calories and 12 grams of protein per serving.

Seitan. Made from wheat gluten, seitan has a decidedly meaty taste and texture. It's available in refrigerated, pre-made form, or in dry form to be prepared at home. Seitan is a great chicken and beef substitute, with a more convincing texture and taste than most other meat substitutes. Generally, it weighs in at about 100 calories and 15 grams of protein per serving.

Burgers and more. Most "vegetarian burgers" are made from soy protein and may contain other beans, as well as grains and vegetables. They come in many flavors, shapes, and sizes, with low-fat and fat-free versions, and are a convenient protein source. They range from 100 to 170 calories and 10 to 15 grams of protein per serving.

Non-Dairy Milks[29]
(8-ounce serving)

	Skim milk	Soy (low-fat)	Rice	Almond	Multigrain
Calories	85	100	120	70	150
Fat (grams)	0.3	2.5	2	2.5	2
Cholesterol (mg)	5	0	0	0	0
Sodium (mg)	125	90	90	100	50
Protein (grams)	8	5	1	2	3
Calcium (mg)	300	280	280	20	150
Vitamin A*	10%	10%	10%	0%	0%
Vitamin C*	4%	0%	25%	4%	0%
Iron*	0%	8%	0%	0%	0%
Vitamin D*	25%	30%	25%	0%	0%

*Refers to percentage of Daily Value based on 2,000 calorie diet

Milk. Soy milk is the creamiest alternative, and rice milk is a lighter, sweeter option. Soy milk has about 80 calories per cup, with 5 grams of protein. Non-fat soy milk has a nutritional lineup comparable to skim milk. Rice milk has a similar lineup to soy milk, with slightly higher calories. Grain, nut, and seed milks are other options. Most are available in low-fat and calcium-fortified versions. Chocolate and vanilla flavors are available as well.

Cheese. Cheese alternatives made from soy, rice, nuts, and seeds come in a range of flavors, from mozzarella and cheddar to cream cheese and Parmesan. Many contain casein milk protein, so they're not appropriate for people with serious milk allergies. Soy cheddar and mozzarella cheese alternatives have about 80 calories per ounce, 4 grams of fat and 6 grams of protein. Grain, nut, and seed cheeses are lower in fat and calories.

Non-Dairy Cheeses[30]
(1-ounce serving)

	Calories	Fat (grams)	Protein (grams)	Calcium (mg)	Sodium (grams)
Soy cheddar	80	5	6	200	280
Tofu Jack, fat-free	40	0	7	200	240
Almond mozzarella	70	3.5	6	100	280
Rice cheese, American	55	2.5	5.5	200	290

Vegetarian Diet Pyramid

So common (and encouraged) are vegetarian diets that The American Dietetic Association (ADA) recognizes a vegetarian diet pyramid, created by the Oldways Preservation and Exchange Trust, a think tank for food issues based in Cambridge, Massachusetts.

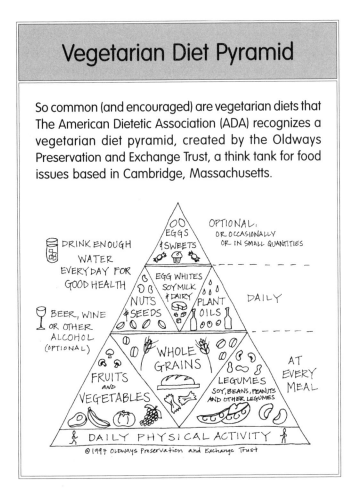

Butter. Most margarines aren't good alternatives for butter, since they contain harmful trans-fatty acids. Butter-like spreads, made from unhydrogenated flax, olive, and other heart-healthy oils, are available at health food stores. They have about 80 calories and 10 grams of fat per tablespoon.

Textured Vegetable Protein. Made from soybeans, textured vegetable protein (TVP) comes in granules, chunks, and flakes. It's great in stews, casseroles, and chili, and can be used as the base for homemade veggie burgers. TVP has about 100 calories and 12 grams of protein per 4-ounce serving.

Fats & Oils...

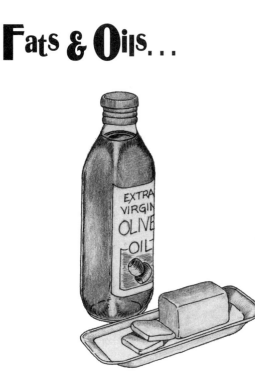

It's the food group we love to hate. High-fat diets have been implicated in heart disease and cancer, and blamed for the nation's widespread weight problems. But lumping fats together in one category is misleading. Some high-quality fats and oils are nutritionally necessary. For instance, the body needs fatty acids to synthesize hormones, make fat-soluble vitamins available to the body, and maintain cell membranes. Stored fat, as much as we hate the sound of it, surrounds and protects organs, provides an accessible source of energy, and acts as an insulator to keep the body warm. The key is in getting the right amount and kinds of fats.

How Much Is Enough?

The American Heart Association recommends no more than 5 to 8 servings of fats and oils per day, depending on caloric needs. (The AHA advises limiting fat intake to 30 percent or less of total calories.) Nuts, seeds, olives, and avocado are included as fats in the USDA's Food Guide Pyramid. A serving is equivalent to about 1 teaspoon of fat. Some examples:

✗ 1 teaspoon of olive oil
✗ 2 teaspoons of peanut butter
✗ a small handful of nuts
✗ one ½-inch thick slice of avocado
✗ 5 large olives

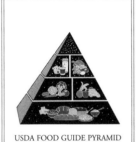

USDA FOOD GUIDE PYRAMID

Shopping and Storage Tips

Choose fats and oils carefully. Monounsaturated fats—those found in cold-pressed, extra-virgin olive oil, canola oil, and some nut oils—are the best choices. Use butter in moderation. Avoid saturated vegetable oils (palm oil, coconut oil). Keep in mind that most margarines are made with hydrogenated oils and contain trans-fatty acids, implicated in heart disease risk. Softer margarines contain fewer trans-fatty acids, and some margarines (those made without hydrogenated oil) contain none. New "cholesterol-lowering margarines"—made, for example, with sterols extracted from soybeans—may be a healthy option.

Read labels of processed food for total fat content, and choose processed foods made with unhydrogenated oil rather than hydrogenated or saturated fat.

Store oils in the refrigerator to prevent them from going rancid. They may turn cloudy, but this won't affect their taste or nutrient content.

Oil Change: A Big Fat Controversy

Before you change your oil, read this: studies are showing that all vegetable oils aren't equal, and that margarine isn't necessarily better than butter. Make a healthy oil change by substituting extra-virgin olive oil or canola oil for other vegetable oils, and going very easy on the butter—*and* the margarine, especially stick varieties. More facts on fats:

Saturated fatty acids account for most of the fat in butter, animal products like meat and cheese, and palm and coconut oil. They're usually solid at room temperature. Saturated fatty acids, well-known for their role in heart disease, elevate cholesterol levels and promote atherosclerosis. Their role in cancer is less clear, but they have been linked to breast and colon cancer.[1]

Monounsaturated fatty acids are found in olive oil, canola (rapeseed) oil, nut oils, avocados, olives, almonds, peanuts, pecans, macadamias, and cashews. Monounsaturated oils are liquid at room temperature but begin to solidify when refrigerated. They are considered the most heart-healthy oils, and have been shown to lower cholesterol levels and reduce the risk of cardiovascular disease.[2]

Canola oil, made from rapeseed, is nutritionally similar to olive oil. One important difference: it's higher in alpha-linolenic acid, which the body converts into omega-3 fatty acids, known for their role in protecting against heart disease and other chronic illnesses. In fact, recent data from the Lyon Diet Heart Study suggests that canola oil may be a key factor in the low rate of heart attacks among those who eat a traditional "Mediterranean diet."[3]

Polyunsaturated fatty acids are abundant in corn oil, safflower oil, sunflower oil, soybean oil, and walnuts. They are liquid at room temperature and stay liquid when refrigerated. Because they easily combine with oxygen, polyunsaturated oils can become rancid very quickly and must be kept refrigerated. They're considered heart-healthy, but their role in cancer is less clear. Study results conflict, for example, on a possible association between polyunsaturated fat consumption and breast cancer risk.[4] Two types of polyunsaturated fats— omega-3 and omega-6 fatty acids—are of particular interest for their role in protecting against heart disease, cancer, stroke, and diabetes.[5] (See pages 165–166.)

Trans-fatty acids are found in most kinds of margarine, hydrogenated oils, and many processed foods, including cookies and white bread. They are created during hydrogenation, a process used to make liquid fats solid, as in the case of margarine, or to extend the shelf life of fats used in processed foods. When unsaturated fatty acids are hydrogenated, a chemical change occurs in which the fatty acids become saturated. Studies have shown that trans-fatty acids and hydrogenated fats raise total blood cholesterol levels, increase harmful LDL cholesterol, decrease beneficial HDL cholesterol, and increase lipoprotein(a)—any of which can contribute to cardiovascular disease.[6]

Compared to harder processed fats like stick margarine, butter, and lard, softer fats such as tub margarine and oil tend to have fewer trans-fatty acids. Research from the USDA's Nutrition Center at Tufts University in Boston, reported in the *New England Journal of Medicine* in June 1999, shows that softer fats have better effects on blood levels of LDL and HDL cholesterol.[7]

Essential Knowledge: The ABCs of EFAs

The best of the good fats, essential fatty acids (EFAs) are crucial for good health. EFAs are responsible for regulating prostaglandins, the hormone-like chemical messengers that help transport oxygen and control pain, blood pressure, and inflammation. EFAs also aid in maintaining cell membranes and transporting waste and nutrients in and out of cells. The potential role of EFAs in reducing the risk of cancer, heart disease, and other illnesses have made them one of the nutritional darlings of the '90s.[8, 9]

Since the body can't manufacture EFAs, they have to come from food sources. The two families of EFAs are:

✗ Omega-3 (alpha-linolenic) fatty acids, abundant in cold-water fish like salmon, mackerel, tuna, and trout, and in dark leafy greens, flaxseed, walnuts, and canola oil. (See "The Fatted Fish," page 125.)

✗ Omega-6 (linoleic) fatty acids, found primarily in vegetable oils.

The typical American diet is higher in omega-6 than in omega-3 fatty acids. This can be problematic. Omega-3 and omega-6 fatty acids should occur in a balanced ratio of 1:1, because an excess of omega-6 fatty acids can be harmful. Omega-6s in excess can promote cancer cell proliferation,[10, 11] while omega-3s inhibit it.[12] Low levels of omega-3s relative to omega-6s may also increase the risk of diabetes.[13]

The good news is that a whole-foods diet can create a healthy balance between the two EFA families. For this purpose, regular consumption of dark leafy greens and cold-water fish are highly advised. Some quick ways to up omega-3 intake: drizzle flaxseed or canola oil on steamed greens, sprinkle chopped walnuts on salads and oatmeal, and buy cereals and breads that contain flaxseed.

Fat Stats:
About Cholesterol

There's good cholesterol, and there's bad cholesterol. And how much is too much, anyway? Here is some vital information on cholesterol.

Cholesterol. Cholesterol is a steroid—the most abundant steroid in human tissues. It has important functions in the body, including the production of hormones and the formation of cell membranes. The body manufactures all the cholesterol it needs, yet we get more of it from foods. It is present only in foods of animal origin. Plant foods contain no cholesterol.

It was long thought that high-cholesterol foods increased blood cholesterol. But research in recent years has shown that saturated fat has a greater effect on increasing cholesterol, leading to increased risk of cardiovascular disease and possibly added cancer risk as well.[14, 15] To reduce health risks, total blood cholesterol should be less than 200 milligrams per deciliter of blood.

Lipoproteins. Because cholesterol is fat-soluble, it is unable to dissolve in the blood, so it attaches to proteins to form compounds known as lipoproteins, which carry it around the body. There are several types of lipoprotein cholesterol compounds, including LDL and HDL cholesterol.

LDL cholesterol. LDL (low-density lipoprotein) takes cholesterol to the tissues. High levels of LDL promote a build-up of plaque in the artery walls—hence the name "bad cholesterol." LDL cholesterol should be less than 130 mg per deciliter of blood.

HDL cholesterol. HDL (high-density lipoprotein) carries cholesterol to the liver to be processed and excreted. Because high levels of HDL cholesterol discourage the build-up of plaque in the artery walls, it's known as "good cholesterol." HDL blood cholesterol levels should be above 35 mg per deciliter.

The ratio of total cholesterol to HDL cholesterol is also important, since it is a single measure indicating whether cholesterol is being deposited into the arteries or taken to the liver to be excreted from the body. It is calculated by dividing total cholesterol by HDL (e.g., $200 \div 5$ = a 4:1 ratio). A ratio of 5:1 or lower is considered desirable.

Lipoprotein(a). Recently, a compound known as lipoprotein(a) or Lp(a) has been found to be a risk factor for heart disease. When Lp(a) blood levels are above 30 mg per deciliter, the risk of heart disease is increased.[16]

The Skinny on Fats: How Low Can You Go?

Once researchers noted the dangers of a high-fat diet, the American public jumped on the fat-free bandwagon. When subsequent research pointed out the beneficial effects of certain fats, like those found in olive oil, fish, and walnuts, experts reconsidered the fat-free approach. The American Heart Association now warns that restricting fats to less than 15 percent of total calories can increase triglycerides and lower beneficial HDL cholesterol levels. There is also recent evidence that, in

Foods That Affect Cholesterol Levels[17]

...for better...	...for worse...
Fruits and vegetables	Fatty red meats, processed meats, and organ meats
Whole grains	Cheese
Beans and peas	Whole milk, cream, ice cream
Olive oil	Butter and margarine
Olives	Egg yolks
Canola oil	Bakery items made with saturated fats
Safflower oil	Saturated oils (coconut, palm)
Walnuts and almonds	Snacks with hydrogenated oils (e.g., potato chips, cookies)

terms of heart health, adding polyunsaturated fats may be as important as reducing saturated fats.[18]

On the flip side: One study showed that people with existing coronary heart disease who followed American Heart Association diet guidelines had *twice* as many heart attacks, bypass surgeries, and other coronary events during a five-year study than those who followed a program created by Dr. Dean Ornish, Professor of Medicine at the University of California, San Francisco. The program includes a vegetarian diet that allows 10 percent of calories from fat, and excludes saturated fats.[19] Yet this diet is very difficult for most Americans to follow. And as noted, it may bring its own risks.

Fake fats: too good to be true?... If it sounds too good to be true, it probably is. Fat-fearing Americans were ready for the introduction of Olestra, a non-caloric dietary fat substitute made by esterifying sucrose with fatty acids from edible oil. It is not absorbed or metabolized, so it has no impact on cholesterol levels. Olestra is used in a number of snack foods, including Wow!® potato chips. It is listed as Olean® on food labels.

Concerns have been raised by consumer groups and the medical community about negative side effects of Olestra, including intestinal cramping, diarrhea, flatulence, and other gastrointestinal effects.[20] But in a study reported in the *Journal of the American Medical Association,* researchers found no differences in the gastrointestinal effects of eating potato chips containing Olestra or regular potato chips.[21] Olestra has also been shown to cause a decrease in absorption of fat-soluble vitamins, including vitamin E,[22] and in carotenoids.[23] On the other hand, foods rich in these nutrients are rarely consumed with Olestra snack foods, while some Olestra foods have been fortified with these nutrients.

Overall, moderate consumption of foods containing Olestra appears to be safe. Just keep in mind that fat substitutes are not license to overeat.

Herbs & Spices...

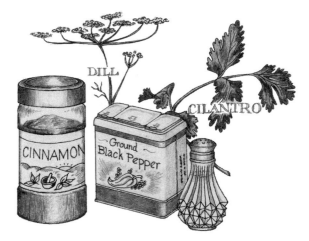

Cutting down on fat and salt in cooking doesn't mean being condemned to a bland diet. Herbs and spices are the best way to add flavor to foods, without adding fat, cholesterol, or sodium. Not only do fresh and dried herbs and spices offer a variety of tastes while containing few calories and no fat—many are sources of healthy phytochemicals and healing compounds. Parsley and cilantro, for example, are high in beta carotene and potassium. Parsley and dill are concentrated sources of lutein and zeaxanthin, antioxidants associated with prevention of vision problems.

Here's an overview of herbs and spices, and how to use them in healthy meal planning.

Shopping and Storage Tips

Choose fresh, whole herbs that are bright green and tender. Avoiding those that are wrinkled, spotted, or browning. Select dried herbs that still have a green hue—those that are brownish are usually very old.

Dried herbs and spices will keep longest if stored in a dark cupboard, away from light, heat, and moisture (storing them on a spice rack above the stove is the *worst* place).

Parsley, Sage, Rosemary, and More

Don't get stuck in the parsley rut. An enormous variety of herbs and spices, both fresh and dried, offer lots of alternatives for every taste imaginable. A brief glossary follows.

Allspice. Used in pumpkin pie, pickled foods, cookies, and cakes. Tastes like a combination of cinnamon, nutmeg, and cloves.

Anise. Has a licorice-like flavor. Used in shrimp and crab dishes, cookies, and cakes.

Basil. Use fresh or dried in soups, stews, salads, and sauces. Especially good with tomato and tomato dishes. Rich and sweet, with a slightly anise-like flavor.

Bay leaf. Has a pungent, fragrant flavor and aroma. Used whole to season cooking soups and stews. Remove whole leaf before serving.

Caraway seed. Has an anise-like flavor. Traditionally used in rye breads and crackers.

Cardamom. Has a rich, sweet and fragrant flavor. Used in curries and Indian food, and in breads, cookies, pastries, and teas.

Cayenne. Hot and spicy, used in chili, Mexican dishes, and any dish that needs a pungent bite.

Celery seed. Has a strong celery flavor. Good in fish dishes, salad dressing, and soups, stews, potato salad, and salad dressing.

Chervil. Pungent, with a distinctive "green" flavor. Can be used like a stronger parsley, in eggs, fish dishes, and sauces.

Chives. Have a mild onion flavor and aroma. Good in salads, egg dishes, potatoes, sauces, and salad dressings.

Cilantro. Often called Chinese parsley, has a distinctive, earthy and musky flavor. Used in Mexican, Chinese, and Thai cooking, and in salads, egg dishes, sauces, soups, stews, meat dishes, and vegetable dishes.

Cinnamon. Sweet, rich and aromatic. Used in cookies, pies, breads and pastries, in some vegetable dishes, sauces, and curries, and in pickling.

Cloves. Strong, sweet and pungent, used in cookies, breads and pastries, soups, stews, ham dishes, and cooked fruit dishes.

Coriander. From the seeds of the cilantro plant. Aromatic and distinctive, with a flavor reminiscent of citrus and sage. Used in curries, cookies, cakes, breads, pastries, and some vegetable dishes.

Cumin. A very strong, earthy and musky flavor, used in Mexican dishes, soups and stews, and vegetables.

Dill. Pungent and sharp, used in pickling, and for soups, sauces, eggs, and potato dishes.

Garlic. Strong and spicy, used in nearly any vegetable, meat, fish, egg, or other dish.

Ginger. Slightly sweet and spicy, with a pronounced bite. Especially associated with Chinese and Japanese cooking. Used in curries, marinades, chutneys, pickles, cookies, cakes, breads, and pies.

> Many herbs and spices contain potent, health-protective antioxidants. Here are some of the most common: parsley, cilantro, rosemary, dill, allspice, clove, cumin, mustard seed, saffron, turmeric, and curry leaf.

Mace. Sweet and fragrant, commonly used in combination with cinnamon, nutmeg, and clove in cookies, cakes, pies, and breads.

Marjoram. A slightly woody, delicate flavor, used in stuffings, egg dishes, game dishes, soups, and stews.

Mint. Aromatic and slightly sweet, traditionally used in pea soup and with lamb dishes, and to flavor fruit, salads, and vegetable dishes.

Nutmeg. Bittersweet and pungent. Used in egg dishes, custards, and fruit dishes, and with cinnamon and clove in baking.

Oregano. A slightly sweet, pine-like flavor. Good in tomato dishes, soups and stews, and meat or fish dishes.

Paprika. Often used for its brilliant red-orange color in rice dishes or as a garnish for broiled fish, potato salads, and other vegetable dishes.

Parsley. With a mild, delicate "green" flavor, used as a garnish and in vegetables, soups, eggs, and meat dishes.

Pepper, black. Pungent, spicy and hot, used in cooking and as seasoning after cooking for vegetables, meats, soups, sauces, and stews.

Pepper, white. Made from black peppercorns with the dark outer hull removed. Slightly less pungent, used in cooking rather than at the table. Also used in white sauces and gravies, when the color of pepper isn't desirable.

Rosemary. Fragrant, green, and piney flavor, used for poultry and meat dishes, sauces, soups and stews, and in salads and vegetable dishes.

Saffron. A very mild and expensive spice prized for its brilliant orange color and delicately earthy flavor. Used in curries, rice, and chicken dishes, and in some baking. Turmeric is often substituted because of cost.

Sage. Strong and fragrant, used in stuffings, with poultry and eggs, and in soups, stews, and vegetable dishes.

Tarragon. With a subtly anise-like flavor, used in egg and vegetable dishes, and to flavor sauces, salad dressings, soups, and stews.

Thyme. Has a fresh, delicate flavor. Good in sauces, soups and stews, stuffing, vegetable dishes, and poultry dishes.

Turmeric. Yellow in color and mild in flavor, adds a golden hue to curries, sauces, rice dishes and baked goods. Often used instead of saffron.

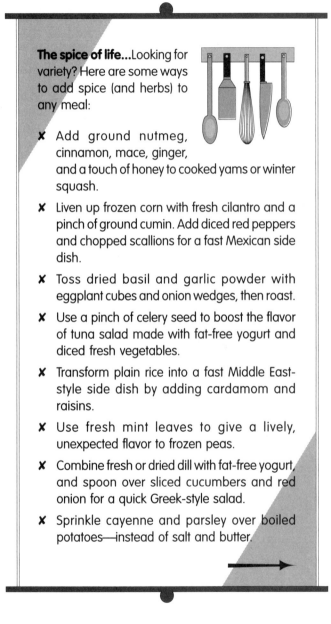

The spice of life... Looking for variety? Here are some ways to add spice (and herbs) to any meal:

✗ Add ground nutmeg, cinnamon, mace, ginger, and a touch of honey to cooked yams or winter squash.

✗ Liven up frozen corn with fresh cilantro and a pinch of ground cumin. Add diced red peppers and chopped scallions for a fast Mexican side dish.

✗ Toss dried basil and garlic powder with eggplant cubes and onion wedges, then roast.

✗ Use a pinch of celery seed to boost the flavor of tuna salad made with fat-free yogurt and diced fresh vegetables.

✗ Transform plain rice into a fast Middle East-style side dish by adding cardamom and raisins.

✗ Use fresh mint leaves to give a lively, unexpected flavor to frozen peas.

✗ Combine fresh or dried dill with fat-free yogurt, and spoon over sliced cucumbers and red onion for a quick Greek-style salad.

✗ Sprinkle cayenne and parsley over boiled potatoes—instead of salt and butter.

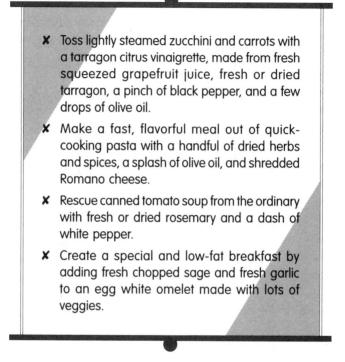

✗ Toss lightly steamed zucchini and carrots with a tarragon citrus vinaigrette, made from fresh squeezed grapefruit juice, fresh or dried tarragon, a pinch of black pepper, and a few drops of olive oil.

✗ Make a fast, flavorful meal out of quick-cooking pasta with a handful of dried herbs and spices, a splash of olive oil, and shredded Romano cheese.

✗ Rescue canned tomato soup from the ordinary with fresh or dried rosemary and a dash of white pepper.

✗ Create a special and low-fat breakfast by adding fresh chopped sage and fresh garlic to an egg white omelet made with lots of veggies.

In a Pinch: Substituting for Salt

The harmful effects of a high-sodium diet are well known. In people who are "sodium sensitive," an excess of sodium can lead to edema, kidney problems, hypertension, heart disease, even stomach cancer.[1,2] The American Heart Association recommends that healthy individuals limit sodium intake to no more than 2,400 mg per day, compared to the current national

average of 3,000 to 4,000 mg. The "DASH Diet"—
Dietary Approaches to Stop Hypertension, endorsed by
the National Heart, Lung, and Blood Institute—
recommends a maximum of 3,000 mg of sodium a day.

Salt of the earth...or salt of the sea? Which is better? Most salt is mined and refined, removing the more than 70 different naturally-occuring minerals like iodine. Natural sea salt, available at natural food stores and some specialty markets, contains all these minerals as they occur in seawater. Commercial refined salt uses chemicals and extremely high temperatures to remove naturally-occuring minerals in salt and refine it to pure sodium chloride. There is some indication that sea salt is better utilized by the body.[3] Because of this, however, some people with poor kidney function must be careful not to overdo it with sea salt.

Many Americans have learned to use less salt in cooking and at the table. Yet about 75 percent of the sodium we consume comes from processed foods.[4] Some packaged foods are extremely high in sodium. For example, 1 cup of rice from a boxed mix may contain up to 1,600 mg of sodium, more than half of the maximum amount recommended. A cup of a popular brand of chicken noodle soup contains 1,169 mg of sodium—more salty than a fast-food hamburger.

Furthermore, we often eat sodium by other names—it's ubiquitous and often well-hidden in common foods. Sodium chloride and sodium nitrate are obvious examples. Some others: calcium disodium, carrageenan (sodium carrageenan), disodium phosphate, monosodium glutamate (MSG), trisodium citrate, and trisodium phosphate.

Labeling can be tricky. "Sodium-free" or "very low sodium" descriptions can be taken literally, but terms like "reduced-sodium" are relative. Reduced-sodium chips, for example, may have less salt than regular chips, but they can still pack a salty punch. Salt watchers are not even safe with foods labeled unsalted or no salt added, since they may contain other sources of sodium, like those listed above.[5]

Luckily, herbs and spices are great alternatives to salt. It's a good idea to keep several varieties on hand to use in a pinch. Still, don't neglect to check labels carefully—many herb and spice seasoning mixtures are actually made with salt. Some tips:

✗ Look for salt-free seasonings made with herb and spice mixtures.

✗ Fill a peppermill with whole mustard seeds, and add a couple of grinds to foods during cooking. (Don't use ground mustard at the table—uncooked, the flavor is harsh.)

✗ "Lite" salt blends contain a mixture of table salt and potassium chloride, for half the sodium. Some are nearly all potassium chloride, and may upset mineral balances. Check with a health care professional first.

✘ Rediscover pepper. Invest in a good grinder and try pink, green, white, and black peppercorns (combined, if you like).

✘ Make several custom blends of favorite dried herbs and spices for different uses. Keep them near the stove and add during cooking. Good choices: tarragon, thyme, sage, chives, oregano, basil, and rosemary.

Healing with Herbs and Spices

Herbs and spices have been used for centuries for medicinal and culinary purposes. Below are some examples, with highlights of traditional healing uses and findings from modern research.

✘ **Cayenne pepper** is traditionally used to ease pain from muscle stiffness, inflamed joints and arthritis, and to treat headaches. It may also help lower cholesterol levels, fight heart disease, and reduce the risk of cancer.[6]

✘ **Cilantro** is used to promote digestion, ease stomach pains, and as an antiseptic, to prevent infection. It may also help relieve arthritis pain.[7]

✘ **Cinnamon** has been used medicinally for thousands of years to prevent infection, soothe upset stomach, prevent ulcers, and control blood sugar.[8]

✘ **Dill** is used to prevent flatulence and aid digestion. It is also a natural preservative, inhibiting the growth of several bacteria including E. coli, which is why it was originally used in pickling vegetables.[9]

✗ **Garlic** is perhaps the oldest traditionally-used medicinal and culinary herb. Modern research shows it can help decrease cholesterol levels, prevent blood from clumping and sticking to artery walls, and reduce the risk of cancer.[10, 11]

✗ **Ginger** is known for its ability to soothe upset stomachs, reduce nausea, and ease motion sickness. It also eases digestion by virtue of its compounds that are similar to digestive enzymes in the stomach.[12] In addition, it may reduce blood platelet clumping and provide some protection against heart disease.[13]

✗ **Oregano** has been use for centuries to treat cuts, bruises and muscle pain, and to relive flu-like symptoms including fever, vomiting, and diarrhea. It is used in herbal medicine for digestive complaints and minor coughs.

✗ **Parsley** is a traditional herb for freshening breath and boosting digestion. It's also used as a diuretic, and to reduce urinary tract inflammation and facilitate the passage of kidney stones.[14]

✗ **Rosemary** has been used to treat menstrual disorders and aid digestion. It is often used in food and cosmetics as a preservative and for its antioxidant properties; it may help protect against breast cancer.[15]

✗ **Sage** is a traditional antiseptic, used to prevent infection, reduce inflammation, and help heal skin. It is also used as a gargle for sore throats and to reduce excessive perspiration such as due to hot flashes in menopausal women.

✗ **Tarragon** contains caffeic acid, a possible anti-carcinogenic substance that can fight free radicals and kill some viruses.[16]

✗ **Thyme** contains thymol, an aromatic antiseptic compound used in some mouthwashes and as a chest rub for colds and congestion.

✗ **Turmeric's** active component, curcumin, is a potent antioxidant and anti-inflammatory agent. Found to inhibit the initiation and promotion of malignant tumors, turmeric has been called "an ideal functional food for prevention of cancer."[17]

(*Note*: Individuals should consult a health professional before trying herbal remedies.)

Sugars & Sweeteners...

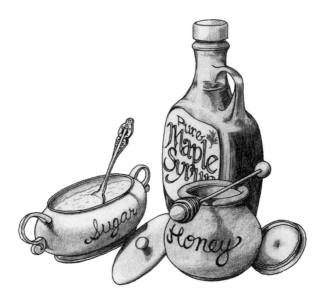

It may be the most comfortably familiar of all food ingredients, but our relationship with sugar teeters between love and hate. Unlike fats, which we've come to universally vilify, sugar makes us sway with indecision, between passion and disdain. Confusion abounds: natural foods enthusiasts shun table sugar in favor of honey and other "natural" sweeteners, yet most of these sweeteners contain sucrose, the same chemical component of white sugar. Artificial, "high-intensity" sweeteners are an alternative, as they are non-cariogenic and non-caloric, though they are not problem-free.

How Much Is Enough?

There is no requirement for refined sugar in the human diet. The USDA and American Dietetic Association advise using sugars in moderation, and sparingly if calorie needs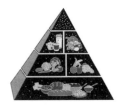

USDA FOOD GUIDE PYRAMID

are low. The Food Guide Pyramid encourages consumers to derive the smallest percentage of their energy from simple sugars.

The Not-So-Sweet Story of Sugar

Americans have a sweet affair with sugar: it is estimated that added sugar makes up about 10 percent of the calories in the average American diet.[1] Processed and packaged foods, ranging from fat-free salad dressings to low-fat crackers, often contain sugar as the second or third predominant ingredient. There are a number of problems with sugar—as well as several common but unproven myths about its health effects.

It is well known, for example, that sugar is cariogenic. Sugar and refined carbohydrates in general cause cavities by interacting with bacteria in the mouth, producing acids that create holes in the tooth's enamel.

Sugar is frequently blamed for obesity, but in and of itself white sugar isn't a high-calorie food. The link between obesity and sweets may have more to do with the fact that high-sugar foods like doughnuts, cakes, cookies, and pastries are also high in fat. The position of the American Dietetic Association is that high-fat foods and too many calories, rather than high-sugar foods per se, are leading causes of obesity.

While refined sugar can be a problem for people with diabetes, there is no evidence that sugar actually *causes* diabetes. Moreover, when eaten by diabetics as part of a meal, a moderate amount of sugar is often tolerated.

Sugar was once thought to increase hyperactivity in children, but the research does not support this theory. And while a number of behavioral disorders—including mood swings, depression, confusion, and fatigue—are sometimes blamed on sugar consumption, research hasn't been able to corroborate these purported effects.[2]

Independent of all this, the main argument against refined sugar is that its role in a healthy diet may be nil. Sugar as a chemical compound provides energy and absolutely no nutrition (with the exception of some "natural" sweeteners that contain trace amounts of vitamins and minerals). All dietary carbohydrates except fiber break down into sugars during digestion, supplying energy and varying levels of nutrients. Rather than depend on sweets for fast energy, it is preferable to rely on nutrient-dense complex carbohydrates like fruits, vegetable, breads, cereals, and grains.

Sweet Nothings:
Natural Sweeteners

Sugar is sugar...almost. Sweetener in any form—honey, fructose, rice syrup—is broken down into glucose in the body. Yet depending on the sweetener, there is a difference in the nutrient content as well as the rate at which glucose is dumped into the bloodstream. Hence, the popularity of sweet alternatives to refined white sugar. Even so, natural sweeteners are highly concentrated and somewhat refined, and are associated with some of the same complaints (cavities, weight gain) that make sugar suspect.

Among natural sugars, brown rice syrup and barley malt have the highest nutrient content and are metabolized more slowly than white sugar, keeping blood sugar on a more even keel for those who are sensitive.

Brown rice syrup, a perennial favorite, has a light but rich flavor. Because it is high in maltose and complex carbs, it's absorbed much more slowly into the blood stream, avoiding the sugar rush and crash. Malted syrups are more expensive but easier on blood sugar levels.

Barley malt syrup has a rich, distinctive taste, similar to molasses. Sprouted barley is used to convert grain starches into a complex sweetener that is metabolized more evenly by the body.

Stevia is a South American herb that's 100 to 400 times sweeter than white sugar. The human body can't metabolize the sweet glycosides in stevia, so it's calorie-free, safe for diabetics, and doesn't cause cavities. Because stevia has a strong, distinctive flavor, however, it's not well-suited to recipes that have a delicate flavor or call for large quantities of sugar.

Fructose comes in granulated and syrup forms and can usually be substituted for white sugar. The crystalline form is almost twice as sweet as white sugar, but it must be converted in the liver to glucose before going into the bloodstream. Because it loses a little of its sweetness when heated, fructose is best used in cold dishes or added after cooking.

Date sugar is a concentrated sweetener from dried and ground dates. It has a grainy texture and a pale brown color, and retains most of the vitamins and minerals found in dates. It can be substituted nicely for brown sugar, but when baking, it may be necessary to reduce oven temperature to prevent excessive browning.

Honey comes in hundreds of varieties, depending on the flower that produces them. Clover and orange blossom are the most popular. Other varieties include alfalfa, buckwheat, heather, linden, raspberry, spearmint, sage, and thyme, all varying widely in taste. Most honey has been pasteurized, which depletes some nutrients. Look for raw, unpasteurized honey (not for children under age two, though).

Maple syrup was used by Native Americans, who boiled down the sap from maple trees and called it sweetwater. Maple sugar, made by boiling maple syrup to evaporate the liquid, is about twice as sweet as white sugar. Some producers use formaldehyde to increase the flow of sap. If this is a concern, look for organic varieties.

Molasses is a by-product of the sugar refining process. The juice from sugar cane and sugar beets is boiled down into a thick syrup, from which sugar crystals are extracted. The "leftover" brownish-black liquid is molasses, which contains the nutrients extracted from sugar cane and sugar beets. Blackstrap molasses amounts to the dregs of the barrel. It's dark and thick, slightly bitter, and contains balancing minerals, including calcium, phosphorous, iron, potassium, magnesium, zinc, and chromium.

Unrefined cane sugar is whole sugar cane in crystal form, with the vitamins and minerals intact. It has a stronger, more distinctive taste than white sugar and is slightly less sweet. It is sold at health food stores.

Brown sugar is simply refined white sugar combined with molasses for a rich taste and soft texture. Because it contains molasses, it also contains small amounts of calcium, phosphorous, iron, and potassium.

Concentrated fruit juice comes in several forms. Fruit concentrates that are evaporated in a vacuum retain vitamins and minerals. By contrast, the most refined forms have virtually no nutrients and their use is linked to high cavity incidence in children. Check the labels.

Artificial Sweeteners

"Non-nutritive" or "high-intensity" sweeteners and products containing them are available for people who want the taste of sweetness but without the calories in natural sugars. Also, unlike "nutritive" sweeteners, high-intensity sweeteners are non-cariogenic and do not produce a glycemic response. Yet there is some controversy about their safety.

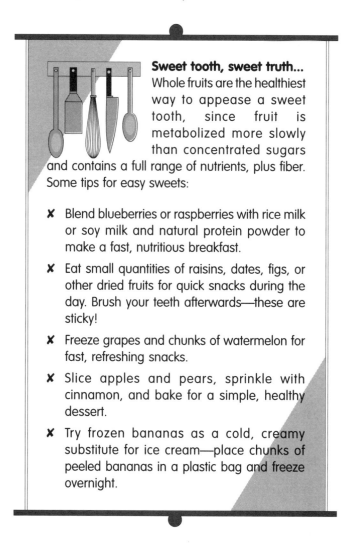

Sweet tooth, sweet truth...
Whole fruits are the healthiest way to appease a sweet tooth, since fruit is metabolized more slowly than concentrated sugars and contains a full range of nutrients, plus fiber. Some tips for easy sweets:

✗ Blend blueberries or raspberries with rice milk or soy milk and natural protein powder to make a fast, nutritious breakfast.

✗ Eat small quantities of raisins, dates, figs, or other dried fruits for quick snacks during the day. Brush your teeth afterwards—these are sticky!

✗ Freeze grapes and chunks of watermelon for fast, refreshing snacks.

✗ Slice apples and pears, sprinkle with cinnamon, and bake for a simple, healthy dessert.

✗ Try frozen bananas as a cold, creamy substitute for ice cream—place chunks of peeled bananas in a plastic bag and freeze overnight.

Ever since saccharin was listed as an "anticipated" human carcinogen in 1981,[3] aspartame has become the artificial sweetener of choice. Acesulfame-K and sucralose are other products in this category approved as food additives by the U.S. Food and Drug Administration. High-intensity sweeteners are used in soft drinks, cereals, chewing gum, and many other products. Depending on the substance, they are 150 to 700 percent sweeter than sucrose.

Aspartame is synthesized from two isolated amino acids which occur in all protein foods. Reported side effects from aspartame include allergic skin and oral reactions and breathing problems.[4] Yet attempts to reproduce these reactions in controlled studies have failed.[5] Other research has explored whether aspartame can cause attention disorders in children,[6] headache, cancer, or brain tumors.[7] These effects are not substantiated, however.

According to the American Dietetic Association, moderate consumption of aspartame and other artificial sweeteners is safe.[8] The American Diabetes Association agrees with the caveat that pregnant or breastfeeding women should not use saccharin and that people with phenylketonuria should not use aspartame.[9] (The latter is a genetic condition in which the body cannot metabolize phenylalanine, one of the amino acids in aspartame.)

The FDA's current position is that people can safely consume 50 mg of aspartame per kilogram of body weight daily over a lifetime without risk. A typical

12-ounce diet soda contains 225 mg of aspartame—so based on this standard, someone weighing 70 kilograms (164 pounds) could consume 3,500 mg, or about 15 soft drinks (or 86 packets of Equal®) per day.[10] (See "Soft Drinks," pages 227–229.)

The long-term effects of artificial sweeteners are unknown.

Deli...

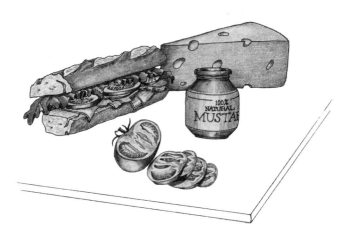

In a perfect world—and a perfect supermarket—the deli section would be a haven for working moms, busy students, anyone who lacks the time, patience, or know-how to cook. In reality, deli foods can be a nutritional nightmare, loaded with fat, cholesterol, and sodium, with little fiber and few whole-food nutrients. Make the wrong choices and you might as well be eating a cheeseburger, fries, and a shake. Still, most deli sections do offer foods that are both nutritious and tasty—including well-chosen sandwiches, phytochemical-rich hot foods and salad options.

Here's a rundown of items offered at the typical supermarket deli, with tips for making healthy choices.

Deli Sandwiches

Prepared sandwiches are a good idea in theory. The problem is that traditional deli meats—ham, bologna, salami—are loaded with fat and cholesterol. Even lean meats like turkey and chicken are packed with sodium in their processed forms. And cheese is high in fat, cholesterol, and sodium.

Portions are another problem: most deli sandwiches use about ¼ to ⅓ of a pound of meat and cheese. Add to that bread and mayonnaise, and classic ham and cheese on rye may weigh in at as many as 800 calories, 47 grams of fat, and 2,100 mg of sodium—more of each than in a Big Mac![1] (Based on 4 ounces of ham, 2 ounces of Swiss cheese, 2 slices of rye bread and 2 tablespoons of mayonnaise.) By contrast, a turkey breast sandwich with 3 ounces of meat and mustard instead of mayonnaise contains only about 300 calories, 5 grams of fat, and 1,000 mg of sodium.

Deli Sandwiches: Healthy Choices

✗ Order turkey breast and chicken breast, ideally in their whole and unprocessed forms for sodium savings.

✗ Ask for half the usual amount of meat on sandwiches, and have the other half wrapped to take home.

✗ Order sandwiches without cheese to slash fat and calories, or get just a quarter of the usual amount.

✗ Substitute mustard or low-fat dressing for mayonnaise. This will save 100 to 300 calories and 10 to 30 grams of fat.

✗ Ask for whole-grain bread. Tortillas or pita bread, if available, are great choices; they have more fiber and fewer calories than white rolls or bread slices.

✗ Request extra tomatoes, onions, lettuce, shredded carrots, or any other veggies available, to boost fiber and phytochemical content.

✗ Even better: if the supermarket has a salad bar, order lean meats and make your own healthy wrap with veggies, pita, and low-fat dressing.

Beware of croissant sandwiches: a 3-ounce croissant has about 20 grams of fat, and that's before counting whatever goes on it.

Hot Foods

Fast, hot food for lunch or dinner is a great idea in theory. But hot foods from the typical supermarket deli leave a lot to be desired. Most are loaded with the usual parade of health villains: fat, sodium, sugars. Vegetables are generally overcooked, over-salted, and prepared with oily sauces and often cheese as well. Worse, deli foods in some stores may languish at lukewarm temperatures for hours, making them a potential breeding ground for harmful bacteria.

Healthy Hot Foods Choices

✗ Construct meals around vegetables. Add rice or potatoes and small portions of lean meats.

✗ Skip the meat loaf and go for chicken breast—and have the skin removed.

✗ Choose whole, unadorned versions of foods: brown rice instead of white, baked potatoes instead of potatoes au gratin. Limit casseroles.

✗ Pick out colorful foods for the highest phytochemical content. Pale or beige foods—meats, casseroles, vegetables in sauce—tend to have more fat and sodium, less fiber, and fewer nutrients.

✗ Combine smaller portions of salty foods with roasted or steamed vegetables to cut sodium while increasing nutrients and fiber.

> A typical deli version of macaroni and cheese is loaded with sodium—some varieties may have as much salt as half a big bag of potato chips.

Prepared Salads

What's in that stuff? Who knows. And since no law requires supermarkets to label prepared foods for fat, sodium, and calories, we can only guess. The only solution is to choose foods that have fairly obvious ingredients. Anything with mayonnaise or creamy dressing is suspect—unless it has been made with low-fat mayonnaise. Food safety is another issue. Deli salads should be well chilled and the case should look scrupulously clean. When in doubt, don't buy.

Deli Salads[2]
(½-cup serving)

	Calories	Fat (grams)	Sodium (mg)
Carrot raisin salad	150	6	340
Chicken salad	250	18	700
Cole slaw, with mayonnaise	170	12	200
Cole slaw, with vinaigrette	110	8	10
Egg salad	245	22	340
Macaroni salad	200	14	360
Potato salad, with mayonnaise	200	14	660
Potato salad, with vinaigrette	150	8	260
Three bean salad	180	8	360
Tuna salad	380	20	820

Prepared Salads: Healthy Choices

✗ Pick vinegar-based salads—such as cucumbers, mushrooms, or peppers in vinaigrette—instead of mayonnaise-based selections, for fat savings.

✘ Cole slaw only looks light. A typical deli cole slaw made with mayonnaise may have at least 40 grams of fat per 2-cup serving, as much as a large shake and fries.

✘ Chicken salad and tuna salad sound healthy. But liberal amounts of mayonnaise make them artery-cloggers. Most have more than 16 grams of fat for a little 4-ounce serving. Choose a skinless chicken breast with honey-mustard sauce or poached salmon with yogurt dill dressing instead.

✘ Practice portion control. Order small servings of oil-based salads, and balance them out with whole-grain bread and a tossed green salad or steamed vegetables.

✘ Boost the fiber and phytochemical content of prepared salads with whole vegetables. Add shredded carrots, beets, or bean sprouts from the salad bar to macaroni salad. Mix extra celery and water chestnuts with tuna salad.

> Surprisingly, deli desserts may not be all bad. Rice pudding, baked apples, and stewed fruits are reasonable in fat content. Even so, fresh fruit is a nutritionally smarter pick.

Salad Bars

The make-your-own salad bar is one of the most brilliant additions to fast food in the last two decades.

Unfortunately, unhealthy offerings at supermarket salad bars can trip up all but the most experienced of customers. It's easy to turn a plateful of healthy, phytochemical-rich vegetables into a goppy, high-fat mess, with oily croutons, bacon bits, nuts, mayonnaise-based items, and salad dressings.

From the Salad Bar: Healthy Choices

✗ Compose salads of fresh, raw veggies for a phytochemical-rich meal, and steer clear of mayonnaise-based salads. The perfect phytochemical salad might include spinach leaves, tomatoes, and carrots, topped with flaxseed oil and vinegar dressing.

✗ Easy on the croutons—one small handful has about 5 grams of hidden fat. Likewise for bacon bits: they are loaded with sodium, about 300 grams in just one tablespoon. For extra crunch, choose water chestnuts or jicama instead.

✗ A handful of nuts can add up to 200 calories and 17 grams of fat to an otherwise healthy salad. Even so, nuts are okay in small amounts (meaning a teaspoon at a time) and they're more nutritious than croutons.

✗ Make wraps or roll-ups with lean meat from the deli and tortillas or pita bread. Load them up with raw veggies and top with fat-free ranch dressing or salsa.

✗ Dressing adds up fast: 2 tablespoons of ranch, blue cheese, or Thousand Island dressing has at least 120 calories and 10 to 15 grams of fat. Mix regular dressing with fat-free dressing or, better yet, cottage cheese, for fat and calorie savings. Other healthy options: vinegar or lemon.

✗ A big bowl of fruit will satisfy a sweet tooth and fruit requirements for the day.

Salad Dressings[3]
(1-tablespoon serving)

	Calories	Fat (grams)	Saturated fat (grams)	Sodium (grams)
Blue cheese	77	8.0	1.5	167
French	67	5.4	1.5	214
Italian	69	7.1	1.0	116
Low-calorie dressings	30-50	1.0-5.0	0-0.5	5-150
Oil and vinegar	70	7.8	1.4	0
Ranch	60	5.0	NA	130
Thousand Island	59	5.6	0.9	109
Balsamic vinegar	10	0	0	0

Bad bugs... Nasty foodborne pathogens cause between 3 million and 12 million cases of foodborne illness and nearly 4,000 deaths every year in the United States. Campylobacter is the leading cause of foodborne infection in the U.S., with an estimated 4 million cases yearly, of which 200 to 1,000 are fatal. It is most commonly traced to contaminated poultry and milk.[4]

Unfortunately, pathogens are more common than we like to think in seemingly innocent foods like rice, fruit, and vegetables.[5] Both E. Coli and salmonella outbreaks, for instance, have been linked to alfalfa sprouts. In 1995, two salmonella outbreaks in the U.S. and Canada sickened about 20,000 people.[6] Foodborne transmission of hepatitis A virus is most common in salads, fruits, vegetables, cold cuts, and sandwiches.[7]

How to protect against foodborne illnesses in the deli section? Buy deli foods and salads only from reputable supermarkets. Make sure hot food is hot and cold food is cold. Ask how recently salads were prepared, and whether they were made on the premises or at off-site locations. And if there's any doubt about a food's safety, return it and notify the manager.

If you become sick and suspect a culprit, contact your local Board of Health. Many cases of food poisoning go unreported.

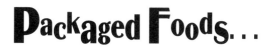

Packaged Foods...

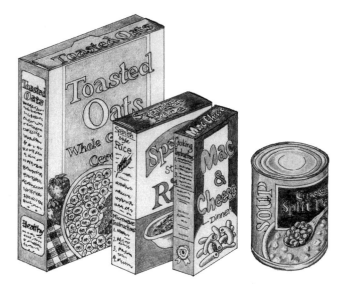

Packaged or processed foods refer to those that are ready to eat, like canned soup, breakfast cereals, and burger mixes. Carefully chosen, they can be a part of a healthy diet. Convenience is a valued commodity, and processed foods from the supermarket can be a healthier choice than, say, drive-through burgers and fries or take-out Chinese. And canned spinach is better than no spinach at all.

Incorporating packaged foods into a health-promoting diet requires some food sleuthing. Food labels can tell the difference between nutritious choices and products that are nutritionally-suspect.

Shopping Tips

Packaged foods vary widely in their nutritional value. The problem with packaged foods involves what has been added during processing, and what has been removed.

Many processed foods, for example, are high in added sodium. Indeed, about 75 percent of all the sodium in the U.S. diet is added during food processing.[1] For example, some brands of canned tomatoes and tomato sauce are high in sodium, while other versions have little or no sodium added. Added sugar is also a concern. Many packaged cereals, canned goods, and beverages are high in sugar, while others are not. Moreover, some canned goods are loaded with artificial flavors, colors, and preservatives, not to mention hydrogenated fats and refined sugars. Others are organic.

Many processed foods have had most or all the fiber removed. This is often the case with cereals made from refined grains. Some canned goods, such as beans, retain most of their nutritional value; others, like canned vegetables, have lost a good deal of their nutrients (such as the water-soluble vitamins depleted due to heating). No one knows for sure how processing affects phytochemicals, but they are thought to be heat sensitive.

From a food smart perspective, many processed foods, altered from their original form, are suspect. Studies on the health benefits of phytochemicals have generally found that whole foods—like fruits, vegetables, whole grains, and legumes—have the most preventive and healing benefits. Dietary recommendations from the

USDA, the American Heart Association, and the National Cancer Institute reflect this perspective.

Following are some examples of healthier choices in packaged foods.

Nut and Seed Butters

Peanut butter can be a quick, relatively healthy snack (high in protein, vitamin E, B vitamins, essential fatty acids, and other nutrients) if spread thinly on whole-grain crackers or apple slices. Watch out for varieties with sugar and added oils (some cheaper brands contain hydrogenated fats). For variety, look for almond butter, sesame seed butter (tahini), and other interesting nut and seed butters.

Nut and Seed Butters[2]
(2-tablespoon serving)

	Calories	Fat (grams)	Fiber (grams)	Vitamin E (I.U.)	Folate (mcg)
Peanut butter	190	16	2	4.8	24
Almond butter	220	18	3	10	21
Cashew butter	210	16	6	0.8	22
Sunflower seed butter	200	16	5	NA	75
Sesame seed butter	210	18	3	1	29
Soy nut butter	170	11	2	NA	NA

Soups

Canned soups make a quick lunch and nearly instant dinner. The biggest culprit is sodium: some varieties have more than half the recommended levels of sodium for an entire day. Many also contain monosodium glutamate (MSG), a flavor enhancer that causes headaches and itching in many people. Buy the low-sodium or sodium-free varieties, and liven them up with herbs and spices. Add noodles, veggies, and canned beans for a heartier meal. And be careful with cream soups, which tend to be high in fat.

Frozen Foods

Frozen foods may offer a healthier option than calling out for sausage and cheese pizza. Individual foods—frozen vegetables, potatoes, and meats—tend to be a better pick, since they have fewer added ingredients and less sodium than complete frozen dinners. Frozen vegetables are better nutritionally than canned varieties.

Canned Beans

Unlike many canned vegetables, canned beans retain most of their original nutrients. They're a high-protein, low-fat starting point for nearly instant meals. Add rice, vegetables (fresh or frozen), herbs and spices for a hearty, fiber-rich meal in minutes.

Breakfast Cereals

Packaged cereals can be a healthier breakfast choice than Danish pastries or muffins, but label scrutiny is indispensable. There's a considerable difference in nutritional value between bright pink, sugar-coated puffs made with refined flour and preservatives and free of fiber, and 100% wheat bran.

Even granola, the once-revered snack of vegetarians, can be a nutritional mistake, loaded with refined white sugar, hydrogenated oils, salt, and preservatives. A ½-cup serving of granola may contain up to 400 calories and 10 to 15 grams of fat (that's without the milk). By contrast, a bran cereal may contain about 100 calories per ½-cup serving, 1 or 2 grams of fat, and double the fiber. (See "The Breakfast Cereal Aisle: Proceed with Caution," page 65.)

Overall, it's better to choose oats or other whole-grain or bran (and sugar-free) cereals. Add a bit of honey, a few walnuts or almonds, fresh or dried fruit, and fat-free yogurt for a healthy breakfast.

Condiments

Salsas, vinegars, relishes, East Indian-style chutneys and pickles, and other highly-flavored sauces can add interest to vegetables, grains, and meat dishes, and are healthier alternatives to fat-based condiments like mayonnaise and sour cream. Another bonus: since they're made with fruits and vegetables, these condiments contain healthy phytochemicals but virtually no fat or cholesterol. Suggestions: spoon chutney over grilled fish, drizzled fruit-flavored vinegar on salads, and top baked potatoes with salsa.

Condiments
(1-tablespoon serving)

	Calories	Fat (grams)	Sodium (grams)
Ketchup	15	0	190
Mayonnaise	100	11	90
Mayonnaise, light	50	5	120
Mustard	0-15	0	180
Chili sauce	20	0	0-360
Sweet relish	20	0	105
Mango lime chutney	50	0	240
Salsa	5	0	85
Red raspberry vinegar	5	0	0
Hot garlic sauce	7	0	215

By the way, fruit preserves are a healthier choice than butter on toast. Combined with vinegar, they make a fast fat-free salad dressing or marinade for chicken or fish. Choose whole-fruit spreads, rather than jams and preserves made with added sugar.

Food Additives: More than Meets the Eye

The food additives industry is huge—at last count, it was worth about $15 billion, with artificial flavors and sweeteners topping the list.[3] It probably comes as no surprise that the United States continues to be the world's biggest market for food additives.

Food additives aren't new. Our ancestors used salt to preserve meats, sugar to lengthen the life of fruit, and vinegar to make cucumbers edible for months. But foods containing synthetic additives—artificial flavors, colors, stabilizers, and preservatives— have little or no place in a whole-foods diet. According to the Food and Drug Administration's Center for Food Safety, several commonly-used preservatives may pose important health concerns. For example:

Nitrites are abundant in bacon, smoked meats, and cured meats. They inhibit the growth of bacterial spores that cause botulism, a deadly foodborne illness. In the body, they may react with secondary amines to form carcinogenic compounds called nitrosamines and nitrosamides. Some government agencies, however, feel that the risk of botulism is greater than the risk of developing cancer from nitrites. Antioxidants such as sodium ascorbate or sodium erythorbate are often used with nitrites to inhibit the formation of nitrosamines.[4]

Butylated hydroxyanisole (BHA) is a phenolic antioxidant used to prevent rancidity of fats and oils. When the food additives amendment was enacted in 1958, BHA was listed with preservatives considered generally recognized as safe (GRAS). Since that time, BHA has been removed from the GRAS list, and studies have suggested that BHA may cause cancer in animals.[5]

Butylated hydroxytoluene (BHT) is a related phenolic antioxidant. Although not toxic itself, BHT may interact with other substances to form carcinogens. BHT has also been removed from the GRAS list.[6]

Sulfites can cause moderate to severe reactions in sensitive individuals. Difficulty breathing is the most common reaction reported; others range from stomach ache and hives to anaphylactic shock. The FDA estimates that one out of 100 people is sulfite-sensitive, and that 5 percent of those with asthma are at risk of an adverse reaction to sulfites. The FDA requires food manufacturers and processors to disclose the presence of sulfiting agents in concentrations of at least 10 parts per million, but the threshold needed to trigger a reaction in a sensitive or allergic person may be even lower.[7] The FDA has banned the use of sulfites on fruits and vegetables intended to be eaten raw, but they may still be included in dried fruits and packaged foods, listed as sulfur dioxide, sodium sulfite, sodium and potassium bisulfite, and sodium and potassium metabisulfite.[8]

Artificial preservatives do add to convenience and cost savings, but aren't really necessary. Some food manufacturers are now using non-synthetic preservatives, such as natural antioxidants like vitamin E, rosemary, and sage. Oil manufacturers are beginning to use ultraviolet-barrier packaging to enhance food preservation. Nitrogen-packed bottles for enhanced stability without preservatives are becoming available.

Nutrition Sleuthing

Studies show that, when it comes to eating habits, knowledge is power. What people know about nutrition is an important factor affecting dietary choices, and people who know more about nutrition tend to have healthier diets.[9] Food labels are an invaluable source of information and a handy tool for making health-promoting eating choices.

New labeling laws enacted in 1994 make it easier to understand food labels. Still, product labels do not tell the whole story, and some contain claims that can be misleading. Moreover, 70 percent of adults surveyed say they would like food labels to be easier to understand.[10] Here are some points to keep in mind:[11]

✘ Most labels list ingredients in descending order by percentage of total volume. For instance, if a cereal has four ingredients, and sugar is the fourth listed, it most likely contains a small percentage of sugar.

Can you guess what this is?...

Ingredients: Unbleached enriched wheat flour [flour, niacin, reduced iron, thiamin mononitrate (vitamin B1)], sweet chocolate (sugar, chocolate liquor, cocoa butter, soy lecithin added as an emulsifier, vanilla extract), sugar, partially hydrogenated vegetable shortening (soybean, cottonseed and/or canola oils), non-fat milk, whole eggs, cornstarch, egg whites, salt, vanilla extract, baking soda, and soy lecithin.

(The food label on page 213 gives the answer.)

✗ "No sugar added" simply means there's no table sugar. There may be other forms of sugar such as corn syrup, dextrose, fructose, glucose, maltose, or sucrose. Check the list of ingredients.

✗ "Calorie-free" indicates less than 5 calories per serving, while "low-calorie" denotes 40 calories or less per serving. "Low-calorie" prepared meals contain 120 calories or less per each 100 grams. "Light or "lite" foods have ⅓ fewer calories or 50 percent less fat compared with what's in a standard serving of the traditional food. A "light meal" is synonymous with "low-calorie" or is "low-fat"—meaning that it has fewer than 3 grams of fat per serving.

✗ "Fat-free" or "100 percent fat-free indicates that the food has less than 0.5 grams of fat per serving, while a "low-fat" food contains fewer than 3 grams of fat per serving. "Reduced-fat" or "less fat" means 25 percent less fat than the standard version of that food. "Saturated fat-free" means that a serving contains less than 0.5 grams of saturated fat and less than 0.5 grams of trans-fatty acids.

✗ Neither "lean" nor "extra lean" necessarily denotes low-fat. "Lean" just means fewer than 10 grams of total fat, no more than 4.5 grams of saturated fat and a maximum of 95 mg of cholesterol per 3-ounce serving. "Extra lean" indicates less than 5 grams total fat, 2 grams saturated fat, and 95 mg cholesterol per serving.

✗ Check serving sizes. Some bottled beverages, for instance, actually amount to 2 servings, which means

Cookies Label

Serving Size reflects the amount typically eaten by many people.

Nutrition Facts

Serving Size 3 cookies (34g/1.2 oz)
Servings Per Container About 5

Amount Per Serving

Calories 180 Calories from Fat 90

% Daily Value*

Total Fat 10g	**15%**
Saturated Fat 3.5g	**18%**
Polyunsaturated Fat 1g	
Monounsaturated Fat 5g	
Cholesterol 10 mg	**3%**
Sodium 80 mg	**3%**
Total Carbohydrate 21g	**7%**
Dietary Fiber 1g	**4%**
Sugars 11g	
Protein 2g	

Vitamin A 0%	•	Vitamin C	0%
Calcium 0%	•	Iron	4%
Thiamin 6%	•	Riboflavin	4%
Niacin 4%			

*Percent Daily Values are based on a 2,000 calorie diet. Your daily values may be higher or lower depending on your calorie needs.

	Calories	2,000	2,500
Total Fat	Less than	65g	80g
Sat Fat	Less than	20g	25g
Cholesterol	Less than	300mg	300mg
Sodium	Less than	2,400mg	2,4000mg
Total Carbohydrates		300g	375g
Dietary Fiber		25g	30g

The list of nutrients covers those most important to the health of consumers.

Calories from Fat are now shown on the label to help consumers meet recommendations that no more than 30 percent of total calories should come from fat.

% Daily Value (DV) shows how a food in the specified serving size fits into the overall daily diet. By using the %DV you can easily determine whether a food contributes a lot or a little of a particular nutrient. And you can compare different foods, with no need to do any calculations.

a double dose of calories and sugars. Snapple® and 16-ounce soft drinks are good examples.

✗ Nutrition Facts information must now include the total amount of fat and saturated fat. But harmful trans-fatty acids are not required to be listed. Mention of hydrogenated oils (or "partially-hydrogenated oils") on the ingredient list indicates that trans-fatty acids are present. It's also useful to know that margarine, cookies, and white bread are among the main sources of trans-fats in the U.S. diet.[12]

✗ A food labeled as "healthy" must be low in fat, saturated fat, cholesterol, and sodium, and, with a few exceptions, must contain at least 10 percent of the Daily Value of vitamin A, vitamin C, iron, calcium, protein, or fiber.

✗ When it comes to food labeling, there is no legally-recognized definition of the world "natural." The term means only that the product has no artificial ingredients or additives—but it may be filled with sugar, fat, or both. A product labeled "natural" is not necessarily a smart food. Remember to read the label!

✗ When the word "natural" is applied to meat, it only means the product is minimally processed and free of additives like sugar, colorings, and preservatives. It does not mean organically-produced meat free of antibiotics and other drugs.

✗ "Natural flavorings" refers to those "derived from a spice, fruit or fruit juice, edible yeast, herb, bark, bud, root, leaf or similar plant material, meat, seafood, poultry, egg, dairy product...whose significant function in food is flavoring rather than nutritional." This broad definition may include such ingredients as hydrolyzed protein, which contains MSG.

Snacks...

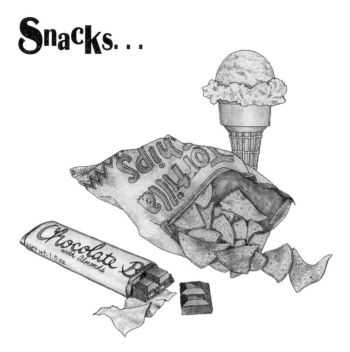

Snacking *can* be part of a healthy eating plan. The best snacks, of course, are whole foods—such as fruit, vegetables, nuts, seeds, dried fruit, and whole-grain crackers. Realistically though, many people will not restrict snacks to apples and carrot sticks. Unbuttered popcorn or rice cakes won't satisfy a hankering for chocolate ice cream or fudge cookies.

The key to healthy snacking is, first, looking for the good ingredients (fiber, vitamins, and minerals) while limiting the bad ones (fat, salt, sugar, and heavy doses of artificial ingredients), and second, choosing healthier, more natural options to high-fat and high-calorie snacks. This chapter presents some alternatives to common snack favorites.

Chips and Pretzels

Baked chips are the best choice. Low-fat chips are another alternative. Look for those made with non-hydrogenated vegetable oils (canola, soybean, sunflower, even olive oil) instead of the bad-for-your-heart hydrogenated variety, and keep an eye on the sodium content.

Chips[1]
(1-ounce serving)

	Calories	Fat (grams)	Saturated fat (grams)	Sodium (mg)	Fiber (grams)
Potato chips	150	10	3	180	1
BBQ potato chips	150	10	3	200	1
Baked potato chips	110	1.5	0	160	2
Fat-free potato chips	75	0	0	260	1
Tortilla chips	140	7	1.5	170	1
Corn chips	150	7	3	180	2
Nacho cheese chips	140	7	1	200	1
Cheese puffs	150	9	2	160	<1
Pretzels	110	1	0	100 -550	2

Most pretzels are fat-free—but many have up to 500 mg of sodium per ounce. Look for salt-free or low-salt versions. Some brands use sesame seeds instead of salt. Whole-wheat varieties are available—with over 2 grams of fiber per ounce, as much fiber as in a medium-sized carrot and nearly as much as in a small apple.

Chocolate

Carob, the sweet, edible pulp from the tropical carob tree, is the most common, but not necessarily adequate, substitute for chocolate. Most carob confections have as much sugar and fat as chocolate. One difference is that, unlike chocolate, carob is caffeine-free. In any case, chocolate has healthful properties (see below) that may warrant its consumption in moderation.

Chocolate may really be the way to our hearts: the stearic acid in cocoa butter (the key raw ingredient in chocolate) may help lower LDL cholesterol levels.[2] Meanwhile, chocolate contains high levels of chemicals known as phenolics, antioxidants which can further reduce the risk of coronary heart disease by preventing LDL cholesterol from oxidizing and clogging the arteries.[3] Not to mention that the polyphenols in chocolate are also known to boost immune function[4]—another reason why eating chocolate in moderation may actually be a healthy habit.

Incidentally, cocoa powder has the same rich chocolate taste but with less fat and fewer calories than milk chocolate.

Chocolate and Carob[5]

	Calories	Fat (grams)	Saturated fat (grams)	Calcium (mg)
Milk chocolate (1.5-ounce bar)	226	13.5	8.0	84
Carob (1.5-ounce bar)	233	13.6	12.7	132
Carob mix, powder (1 tablespoon) with 8 ounces of skim milk	130	0.4	0.3	306
Cocoa mix (1.1-ounce packet) with 8 ounces of skim milk	204	0.4	0.3	402
Chocolate milk, low-fat (8 ounces)	158	2.5	1.5	287
Cocoa powder, unsweetened (1 tablespoon)	12.4	0.7	0.4	7

Cookies

Make cookies count by choosing those made with whole grains. Seeds, nuts, and fruits, instead of artificial ingredients, boost fiber and nutrient content. Look for cookies sweetened with honey, molasses, cane juice, or fruit juice.

Crackers

A wide variety of whole-grain crackers are available, using whole wheat, rice, barley, oats, and other grains. Some have added bran to boost fiber content. Avoid those with hydrogenated oils, and check the sodium content.

Crackers[6]
(14- to 15-gram serving)

	Calories	Fat (grams)	Protein (grams)	Fiber (grams)	Sodium (mg)
Saltines	60	1.5	2.0	<1.0	180
Rye-krisp	60	1.5	1.0	3.0	90
Water	60	1.5	2.0	<1.0	50
Wheat	65	1.5	1.5	0.5	125
Whole-wheat	58	1.3	2.3	1.8	110
Wheat thins	70	3.0	1.0	1.0	90
Melba toast	50	0	2.0	1.0	43
Oyster	60	1.5	3.0	1.0	165
Goldfish	70	3.0	1.5	<1.0	115
Graham	60	1.4	1.0	0.4	86

Herbal hoaxes... In an effort to further woo health-conscious consumers, some snack manufacturers have taken the snacks-can-be-healthy concept to new lengths. Snack foods with names like Personality Puffs (with St. John's wort, the well-known herb for fighting depression) claim to make snackers kinder and happier. Other contenders: kava kava corn chips, valerian chips, and ginkgo biloba corn puffs.

In the unlikely event that any of these snacks do have healing properties, the nutritional expense may not be worth it. A bag of St. John's wort puffs, for example, has 120 mg of St. John's wort. The recommended therapeutic dose of St. John's wort is 900 mg per day.[7] That translates to more than seven bags of chips, and a total of 1,960 calories and 144 grams of fat.

For the time being, it's probably wiser at snack time to stick to a cold, crisp apple, or a low-sodium variety of baked tortilla chips.

Ice Cream

Ice cream and frozen yogurt tend to be high in calories and fats. One nutritional benefit is their calcium content, usually 10 to 15 percent of the Daily Value per ½-cup serving. Most varieties of fat-free ice cream and frozen yogurt pump up the sugar and use gums and other ingredients to maintain the consistency imparted by fat. Natural, low-fat varieties of ice cream, fruit ices, soy milk, and rice milk confections are other frozen snack options.

Frozen Snacks[8]
(½-cup serving or as indicated)

	Calories	Fat (grams)	Saturated fat (grams)	Sugars (grams)
Ice cream	170	9.0	6.0	15
Ice cream, low-fat	100	1.0	0.5	17
Ice cream, no sugar added	99	4.2	2.4	5.7
Sherbet	120	2.0	1.0	25
Sorbet, fat-free	130	0	0	32
Ice milk	110	4.0	2.5	NA
Frozen yogurt	120	4.0	2.0	15
Frozen yogurt, fat-free	100	0	0	20
Frozen juice bar (1 bar)	80	0	0	20
Frozen juice bar, no sugar added	30	0	0	0
Drumstick (1 cone)	300	17	10	21
Fudgsicle	90	1.5	1.0	14
Fudge bar, fat-free	100	0	0	13
Soy frozen dessert	110	1.0	0	14
Rice frozen dessert	150	6.0	0	17

Candy Bars

Natural energy bars tend to be higher in protein, fiber, vitamins, and minerals than candy bars. Some have nearly double the calories, however. Check the labels.

Beverages...

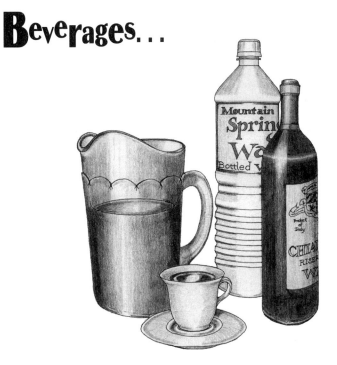

Beverages tend to be an afterthought in most eating plans—they don't *seem* to count—but they can actually make the difference between healthy and so-so diets. (Imagine adding a chocolate shake or a 16-ounce soft drink to an otherwise sensible lunch of tuna salad and whole-grain bread.) Chosen poorly, beverages are a vehicle for excess calories, sugar, fat, artificial flavors, colors, preservatives, even harmful parasites. But if chosen carefully, they can be a nutritious part of any meal plan. For example, water is critical for health maintenance, juices can supply important vitamins and minerals, and green tea is a source of healing phytochemicals.

Some common beverage choices are discussed here. Selections like sweetened, flavored drink mixes, and fruit drinks (as opposed to real juices), have no place in a healthy diet and are not included.

Water

The human body is about 70 percent H_2O, and water is the basis for most beverages. Water is the only beverage that can be consumed in nearly unlimited quantities without adverse health effects. Not only that—drinking water is essential for good health. Unfortunately, recent research suggests that a significant portion of the population may be chronically mildly dehydrated (not surprising considering our national caffeine habit). Dehydration of as little as 2 percent loss of body weight can impair physiological functioning. The research also shows that adequate water consumption can reduce the risk of various illnesses, including childhood and adolescent obesity, urinary stone disease, mitral valve prolapse, and cancers of the breast, colon, and urinary tract.[1]

Based on data showing that water consumption benefits the overall health of the elderly, researchers at the U.S. Department of Agriculture's Human Nutrition Research Center for Aging at Tufts University recommend that people over age 70 drink 8 glasses of water daily.[2] (See page 14.)

The choices for consumers are between tap water and the many varieties of bottled waters available.

There may be reason for concern about drinking tap water. While it is mostly free of bacteria and parasites that will make you sick immediately, many municipal water supplies contain other potentially harmful substances. Some tap water, for example, is high in lead, which leaches from pipes. Tap water also contains chlorine and other chemical additives. Toxic materials like fertilizers, pesticides, and radioactive substances turn up in some water supplies. Flocculents, which make pollutants clump together and are classified as probable carcinogens, may also be present.[3, 4]

In 1996, the Environmental Protection Agency reported that about 10 percent of all community water systems, serving about one of every seven Americans, did not meet standards for tap water treatment or sanitation.[5]

Because the quality of municipal water varies, it's a good idea to find out about the quality and safety of the water supply in your area. This information is available by accessing the Environmental Protection Agency's website at www.epa.gov.

Unless you get a water purifier for your home, bottled water sold in supermarkets is probably safer than tap water. Bottled water comes from a variety of sources. Some products contain calcium and other valuable minerals. On the downside, unlike tap water, most bottled waters are not fortified with fluoride—which may pose significant concerns for dental health.

Spring water is the most common variety. Most are micron filtered and ozonated, and may be treated with reverse osmosis and ultraviolet light as well. Some spring waters and **mineral waters** contain calcium in a highly-absorbable form which research suggests is more available to the body than calcium in dairy.[6] Few contain more than 70 mg of calcium per serving, however.

Distilled water is extremely pure, but the resulting liquid is virtually mineral-free and flat tasting. **Sparkling water** can be naturally occurring, seltzer water, or club soda, and may contain sodium. Most brands don't, and when they do it is a small amount (about 40 to 60 mg per serving), but check the label to be sure.

Best choices: Home-purified tap water, or bottled spring water, reverse osmosis purified water, or sodium-free sparkling water.

Based on a 1999 sampling of bottled water, the Natural Resources Defense Council, an environmental advocacy group, reported that water from 23 of 103 brands tested violated California's limits for some contaminant. Unsafe levels of bacteria, arsenic, and a number of carcinogenic chemicals were among the substances found.[7]

Juices

Made from fruit and vegetables, juices vary widely in their levels of healthfulness. Some packaged drinks look like juices but are actually processed "juice drinks" which contain as much sugar as a soft drink. "Fruit nectars" may contain up to 50 mg of added sugar, although many are also high in vitamin C and other nutrients lacking in sodas.

Best choices: Ideally, fresh, unpasteurized juices would be preferable, but bacteria are a concern. One-hundred percent pure pasteurized juices, without added sweeteners, are an excellent choice; most have lost nutrients added back. They are found in the refrigerated section of supermarkets and grocery stores. Some, such as many varieties of orange juice, are fortified with calcium, adding further nutritional value to existing vitamins and minerals. Remember to add juice into daily meal plans: they count as fruit and vegetable servings. (For more on juice, see "Juicy Details," pages 46–47.)

Soft Drinks

According to a recent report entitled "Liquid Candy: How Soft Drinks are Harming Americans' Health," issued by the Center for Science in the Public Interest, soft drink consumption has doubled in the past 25 years. A generation ago, teenagers drank nearly twice as much milk as soda, but nowadays it's the other way around. These trends may have serious health implications, the report indicates, because of what soft drinks contain and "what they replace in the diet (beverages and foods that provide vitamins, minerals, and other nutrients)."[8]

Soft drinks are loaded with calories (from refined sugar or corn syrup) and artificial flavors and colors, and are completely devoid of nutritional value. Cola drinks are high in phosphorous, in the form of phosphoric acid used as a preservative. This is significant because phosphorous is implicated in the erosion of dental enamel. There is a known link between frequent soft drink consumption ("sipping") and tooth decay. Phosphorous also contributes to calcium loss. Caffeine, present in many soft drinks, further leeches calcium from the body. And in fact, drinking a lot of soft drinks may actually add to risk for osteoporosis.[9]

High-fructose corn syrup is manufactured from cornstarch and contains a high level of fructose. Similar in composition and calorie content to sugar, it is used as a direct and inexpensive substitute for cane sugar when liquid sweeteners are needed, such as in soft drinks. High-fructose corn syrup is also used extensively in other processed foods: jams, jellies, condiments, wine. It is not available for home use.

Diet sodas (accounting for about one-fourth of all soft drink sales)[10] are sweetened with high-intensity sweeteners. (See "High-Intensity Sweeteners," pages 188–191.)

Overall, soft drinks do not fit into a whole-foods diet—and they certainly should not be considered alternatives to water, milk, or juice. Limit consumption to no more than one 12-ounce can per day.

> "Soft drinks provide enormous amounts of sugar and calories to a nation that does not meet national dietary goals and that is experiencing an epidemic of obesity. The replacement of milk by soft drinks in teenage girls' diets portends continuing high rates of osteoporosis. Soft drinks may also contribute to dental problems, kidney stones, and heart disease."
>
> — Center for Science in the Public Interest

Coffee

Americans lead the world in coffee consumption. According to National Institutes of Health figures, four of every five American adults drink at least two 8-ounce cups of coffee per day.[11] The main concern about coffee is its caffeine content—due to caffeine's potential short- and long-term health effects.

About caffeine. Caffeine may improve performance and mood (and help relieve headache pain), but there doesn't seem to be much benefit after the first cup.[12] Significantly, caffeine is a psychologically- and physically-addictive drug.[13] High levels of caffeine consumption have been linked to nervousness, irritability, anxiety,[14] insomnia, stomach upset, and premenstural syndrome.[15] Caffeine is a diuretic, and excessive intake is associated with chronic dehydration[16] as well as increased calcium excretion,[17, 18] bone loss, and osteoporosis.[19]

Knowing beans about coffee... Contrary to popular belief, coffee isn't really a bean at all. It's actually the seed of a "cherry" from an evergreen tree that grows mainly in Latin America, the Caribbean Islands, Africa, the Arabian Peninsula, and Indonesia, in a sub-tropical belt that circles the globe. The coffee plant produces cherries that contain two seeds—what we know as coffee beans. The cherries are picked, and the seeds are removed, roasted, packaged, and shipped to your local grocery store or coffee shop.

The two main types of coffee beans are arabica and robusta. Arabica beans, from altitudes of more than 3,000 feet, are lower in caffeine and produce coffees of superior quality. Robusta beans grow at lower elevations, have more caffeine than arabica beans, and are less expensive—the basic truck-stop variety of coffee.

Roasting procedures dramatically influence the taste of coffee. The longer the roasting time, the more oil is drawn to the surface of the bean, and the fuller the flavor. Lighter roasts usually have a sharper, slightly more acidic taste. Darker roasts have a richer, slightly bittersweet flavor, and are lower in caffeine.

Still, consumed in moderation (250 mg per day), caffeine appears safe for most people.

One cup of drip coffee (that's an 8-ounce *cup*, not a mug) of average strength contains about 150 mg of caffeine. Most coffeehouses offer brews in the Big Gulp equivalent of a cup, which may contain 200 to 400 mg of caffeine. By the way: a shot of espresso actually has less caffeine than a cup of coffee—about 75 mg, approximately half the amount.

> Drinking coffee may help prevent gallstones. In a recent study, men who drank 2 to 3 cups of caffeinated coffee daily over the past 10 years had 40 percent lower risk of symptomatic gallstone disease, compared to those who did not drink coffee regularly.[20]

Best choices: To be prudent, drink no more than 1 cup of caffeinated coffee (or 150 mg of caffeine) per day. Swiss Water Process decaffeinated coffee (in moderation) is a good option. Or, for a coffee-like taste without the caffeine, try brewed or powdered grain beverages made from malted barley and grains, or herbal tea "morning brews" made with chicory.

Coffee should be stored in a cool, dark place, or in the freezer if it is not used within a few weeks.

The Conscious Coffee Generation: Going Organic

Because coffee is grown in tropical regions with lots of bugs, most of it is heavily treated with chemical pesticides. Add to that the chemical solvents used in some decaffeination processes, and an ordinary cup of coffee can be a real chemical brew.

Caffeine Values[21]

	Average caffeine content (mg)
Coffee, brewed, 1 cup (8 ounces)	130
Coffee, brewed, decaffeinated (8 ounces)	4
Coffee, drip, 1 cup (8 ounces)	150
Coffee, drip, decaffeinated (8 ounces)	5
Coffee, instant (8 ounces)	100
Coffee, instant, decaffeinated (8 ounces)	3
Coffee, espresso (2-ounce serving)	75
Coffee, cappuccino (single)	75
Coffee, latte (single)	75
Coffee, mocha (single)	75
Coffee, instant, with chicory (8 ounces)	70
Coffee substitute, cereal grain beverage (8 ounces)	0
Black tea (8 ounces)	80
Green tea (8 ounces)	80
Iced tea (8 ounces)	45
Herbal tea (8 ounces)	0
Cola (12-ounce can)	30–45

As card-carrying members of the coffee generation grew into increased awareness, many of its members became concerned about the stuff in their cuppa joe. In response, a whole crop of natural and organic coffees has sprung up, offering solutions to caffeine and pesticide issues.

Good organic coffees are becoming more widespread and affordable. They are available in health food stores as well as some coffee shops and supermarkets. Buy only decafs using the Swiss Water Process or carbon dioxide (CO_2) decaf methods.

"Swiss Water Decaffeinated" is a patented process that uses only water and no chemicals. Green, unroasted coffee beans are soaked in pure water to draw out both the caffeine and flavor. The beans are then disposed of, and the caffeine- and flavor-saturated water is processed through special carbon filters to remove the caffeine but leave the flavor. After that, another batch of raw beans is soaked in the flavored, caffeine-free water. The water draws out the caffeine, but since flavor agents already saturate the water, no new flavor is drawn from the beans. The resulting beans—free of caffeine and rich in flavor—are then dried and roasted. (The caffeine, by the way, is removed from the water and sold to soft drink manufacturers.) Coffee AG, a Swiss company, holds international patents on this technique.

Tea

Many types of teas exist, and some of them have real health benefits. Teas tend to be lower in caffeine than coffee: about 80 milligrams of caffeine per 8-ounce cup, compared to about 150 mg for coffee.

In spite of the various names, tea is tea. Excluding herbal varieties, all teas come from the tea plant, *Camellia sinensis*. Black, green, and oolong are considered the basic types of teas, but thousands of varieties exist. Variations in flavor, color, and strength are based on factors in growing, harvesting, and processing.

Significantly, research points to the healing benefits of tea. Green tea in particular is a potent antioxidant, and both green and black tea may reduce risk of cancer.[22, 23]

Herbal tea—technically not "tea" at all—became popular in the early 1970s as a healthy alternative to coffee. Chamomile, hibiscus, and other flower blends are still popular. Some brews are used for specific healing purposes: for example, peppermint and ginger for stomach upset, chamomile for relaxation, and senna for its laxative effects.

Bottled "natural teas" with herbal extracts are loaded with refined sweeteners, and the herbs used usually aren't in therapeutic quantities.

Best choices: As noted, green tea may have significant health benefits. Herbal tea—hot or iced, unsweetened, or with a little fruit juice added—is a healthier beverage choice than coffee or soft drinks. (Many herbal teas are not recommended for pregnant or lactating women or children.) To preserve freshness, store tea in a cool, dark place.

A spot of tea through history... The exact origin of tea is unknown, but one romanticized version places it in China with the Bodhidharma, the founder of Zen Buddhism, around 500 AD. According to legend, Ta'Mo', as he was called by the Chinese, had vowed to meditate in a garden near the emperor's palace for nine years. After many years, he closed his eyes one day and fell asleep. Upon awakening, he became so enraged with himself that he sliced off his eyelids and flung them to the ground. They took root in the soil and grew into a tea bush. Thus began the long and illustrious history of tea.

Less fanciful—if not as dramatic—accounts hold that the Chinese emperor Shen Nung actually discovered the tea plant in around 2700 BC. Shen Nung made a point of boiling his water as a matter of health. One day when his servants started a fire to boil his water, some of the leaves from the twigs of firewood blew into the pot. The emperor, intrigued by the fragrant scent of the liquid, tasted the brew and found it palatable. Not long after that, the cultivation of tea began to spread to Japan and the rest of the Far East. Later, tea was brought to Europe by enterprising merchants.

Alcoholic Beverages

Alcoholic beverages fill aisles of most supermarkets, and two-thirds of American adults consume them. The health dangers associated with excess alcohol consumption—such as added risk for obesity, hypertension, heart disease, stroke, liver disease, and fatal automobile accidents—are well-known. When combined with a smoking habit, heavy drinking multiplies risk of lung and some other cancers.

There is evidence that drinking in moderation may have health benefits for some people. Regular consumption of red wine may help explain the relatively low rates of heart disease in Mediterranean countries. Ethanol in all types of alcoholic beverages appears to raise HDL cholesterol and function as an anticoagulant.[24] Antioxidants in red wine (catechins, quercetin, and tannins) have been shown to block oxidation of LDL cholesterol, keep blood platelets from clotting, and help keep blood vessels relaxed—all protective for cardiovascular health.[25, 26, 27] (As of March 1999, red wine can carry a label implying that it has health benefits if consumed in moderation.) These same phytochemicals are also present in grapes and grape juice.

According to many studies, moderate consumption of beer or spirits may be as beneficial as wine.[28]

Best advice. Drink in moderation, if at all. The USDA and the American Heart Association both recommend no more than 1 drink a day for women and no more than 2 drinks a day for men. One drink is equivalent to 12 ounces of beer, 5 ounces of wine, or 1.5 ounces of

80-proof distilled spirit. Any drinking should be done with meals. Those advised not to drink include children, adolescents, women who are pregnant or trying to conceive, people who cannot control their drinking levels, those who are going to drive, and those who use medications that may interact with alcohol.[29]

Food Smart

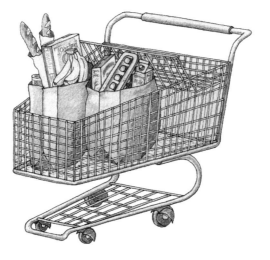

Shopping Cart

Food is food, and medicine is medicine—usually. Yet ever-stronger evidence indicates that certain food groups and specific foods may be considered "nutraceuticals," with proven preventive or healing properties.

As described in these pages, diets rich in fruits and vegetables are associated with lower-than-average incidence of heart disease, cancer, and other chronic, degenerative illnesses. Likewise, diets high in fiber (abundant in plant foods but absent from animal foods) may protect against digestive ailments, blood pressure and cholesterol problems, heart disease, diabetes, and some cancers. Current medical knowledge indicates that including the following foods in the daily diet lowers one's risk of developing health problems:

✗ whole grains

✗ legumes

✗ tomatoes

✗ citrus fruits

✗ soy foods

✗ carrots

✗ grapes and grape products

✗ allium vegetables, such as onions and garlic

✗ orange and yellow fruits and vegetables

✗ cruciferous vegetables, such as broccoli and brussels sprouts

✗ spinach and other dark leafy greens

✗ salmon and other cold water fish

✗ walnuts

✗ almonds

✗ flax

Because of the close interplay between nutrition and disease prevention, consumers have numerous opportunities daily to promote their own good health and well-being.

This can be clearly illustrated by comparing high-fat and low-fat meals.

Sample breakfasts

High-fat	Low-fat
2 fried eggs	Whole-wheat cereal with skim milk
2 sausage links	1 slice of whole-wheat toast with
Danish pastry	1 tbsp peanut butter
Coffee with cream	½ grapefruit
	Coffee with 2% milk

Sample lunches

High-fat	Low-fat
Cheeseburger	Turkey sandwich on whole-wheat
Fries	bread, with mustard
Shake	Green salad with 1 tbsp dressing
	Apple
	Skim milk

Sample dinners

High-fat	Low-fat
Meat and cheese	Baked fish
casserole	Baked potato with 2 tsp butter
Mashed potatoes	Broccoli with lemon
Cauliflower and	Fruit salad with non-fat yogurt
cheddar cheese	Mineral water
Apple pie	
Soft drink	

Nutritional comparisons of these two meal plans are telling:

	High-fat	Low-fat
Calories	2,900	1,900
Fat	185 grams	50 grams
Fat calories	57%	24%
Fiber	10 grams	26 grams
Sodium	4,650 mg	2,000 mg

The low-fat diet is better balanced and more abundant in phytochemical-rich plant foods.

Choosing Wisely in the Supermarket Aisles

The "shopping cart" presented below offers suggestions for making food smart choices. It is organized based on the USDA Food Guide Pyramid, with a few additional categories covered in this book. The lists are not exhaustive, but they do include foods likely to be readily available to most consumers. We encourage health professionals to distribute these guidelines to consumers.

Cereals, Grains, and Bread

Oats, whole-grain cereals, bran cereal, brown rice, bulgur, corn on the cob, polenta, pasta (preferably whole-wheat), whole-wheat bread, multi-grain bread, sprouted-grain bread, pumpernickel, whole-wheat English muffin, corn tortillas, whole-wheat pita, pretzels, baked chips, whole-wheat crackers, low-fat crackers, whole-grain and low-fat cookies, quinoa and other low-gluten grains and breads (especially for gluten-free diets).

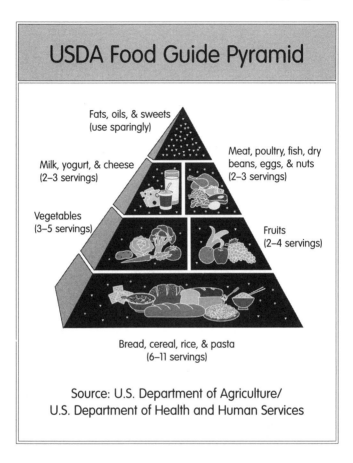

USDA Food Guide Pyramid

Fats, oils, & sweets
(use sparingly)

Milk, yogurt, & cheese
(2–3 servings)

Meat, poultry, fish, dry
beans, eggs, & nuts
(2–3 servings)

Vegetables
(3–5 servings)

Fruits
(2–4 servings)

Bread, cereal, rice, & pasta
(6–11 servings)

Source: U.S. Department of Agriculture/
U.S. Department of Health and Human Services

Vegetables

Onions, garlic, leeks, broccoli, brussels sprouts, cauliflower, radishes, spinach, lettuces, cabbage, kale, chard, mustard greens, carrots, potatoes, sweet potatoes, beets, bell peppers, hot peppers, cucumbers, asparagus, green beans, zucchini and other squash, mushrooms, fennel, parsley and other fresh herbs, fresh salsa.

Fruits

Grapes, oranges, grapefruits, tangerines, bananas, all berries, tomatoes, tomato juice, canned tomatoes, apples, papayas, mangoes, pineapple, cantaloupe, melons, apricots, cherries, peaches, plums, pears, kiwis, persimmons, pomegranates, dried fruits, fresh and chilled juices.

Dairy and Dairy Substitutes

Reduced-fat and fat-free milk, reduced-fat and fat-free yogurt, reduced-fat cottage cheese, Swiss cheese, feta cheese, part-skim mozzarella, part-skim ricotta, fat-free cheeses, soy cheese, soy milk, calcium-fortified rice milk.

Meat, Poultry, Fish, Legumes, Eggs, Nuts, and Seeds

Lean ground beef, round steak, pork loin, veal cutlet, chicken breast (without skin), turkey breast (without skin), game meats (ostrich, buffalo, rabbit, venison), salmon, sardines, trout, tuna, mackerel, swordfish, shrimp, beans, lentils, split peas, peas, tofu, tempeh, miso, eggs, almonds, walnuts, peanuts, cashews, hazelnuts (filberts), pistachios, nut butters, soy nuts, sunflower seeds, sesame seeds, pumpkin seeds, flaxseed, sprouts.

Fats, Oils, and Sweets

Olives, olive oil, canola oil, flaxseed oil, margarine without hydrogenated oil, brown rice syrup, barley malt, molasses, reduced-fat ice cream, reduced-fat frozen yogurt, fat-free sorbet, frozen juice bars, chocolate in moderation, whole-grain cookies, low-calorie natural energy bars.

Deli Choices

Poultry breast sandwiches or lean meats on whole-grain bread, with mustard rather than mayonnaise; vegetable-based hot foods; vinegar-based salads; salad bar salads (fresh vegetables or fruits) with low-calorie or vinegar-based dressing or citrus juice.

Beverage and Snack Choices

Water, juice, green tea, reduced-fat milk, fresh fruits, fresh vegetables, nuts, seeds, baked chips, pretzels, popcorn (not buttered), low-fat crackers, low-sodium crackers, reduced-fat cookies, low-fat frozen desserts.

Balancing Health Concerns with Enjoyment

Being food smart requires making sound food choices based on evolving medical knowledge. But it need not demand self-deprivation or interfere with the pleasure of eating. Consumers should not be discouraged from eating their favorite foods, whatever they may be. A health-promoting diet depends on one's overall eating patterns, on taking advantage of the many nutrient- and fiber-rich foods available today, and on moderating consumption of animal foods, fats and oils, and sweets.

We hope the information in this book will help consumers make sound food shopping and preparation decisions—and develop eating habits which are both health-enhancing and enjoyable.

Appendix...

The tables on the following pages indicate commonly-used recommendations for nutrient consumption.

Daily Values (DV) are reference values currently used as standards on food labels and dietary supplement labels. DVs are derived from two sets of dietary standards, the RDIs and DRVs (see below). "% Daily Value" on labels indicates the proportion of total DV for a given nutrient contained in 1 serving of that food.

Reference Daily Intakes (RDIs) are dietary references based on the Recommended Dietary Allowances (RDAs) for essential vitamins and minerals and, in selected groups, protein. (RDAs are a set of estimated nutrient allowances established by the National Academy of Sciences and updated periodically to reflect current scientific knowledge.) The name "RDI" has replaced the term "U.S. RDA."

Daily Reference Values (DRVs) are dietary references based on a 2,000 calorie diet that apply to nutrients not addressed by the RDAs, including fat, saturated fat, cholesterol, carbohydrates, protein, fiber, sodium, and potassium.

Daily Reference Values (DRVs)*

Food Component	DRV
Fat	≤ 65 grams
Saturated fatty acids	≤ 20 grams
Cholesterol	≤ 300 mg
Total carbohydrates	≤ 300 grams
Fiber	≥ 25 grams
Sodium	≤ 2,400 mg
Potassium	≥ 3,500 mg
Protein**	≤ 50 grams

*Based on 2,000 calories a day for adults and children over age 4.

**The DRV for protein does not apply to certain populations. Reference Daily Intake (RDI) for protein has been established for these groups: Children ages 1 to 4—16 g; Infants under 1 year old—14 g. Pregnant women—60 g; Nursing mothers—65 g.

DRVs for macronutrients and fiber are calculated as follows:

Fat—based on 30 percent of total calories.
Saturated fat—based on 10 percent of calories.
Carbohydrates—based on 60 percent of calories.
Protein—based on 10 percent of calories.
Fiber—based on 11.5 g of fiber per 1,000 calories.

DRVs for cholesterol, sodium, and potassium are always the same, regardless of calorie intake.

Reference Daily Intakes (RDIs)

Nutrient	Amount
Vitamin A	5,000 I.U.
Vitamin C	60 mg
Vitamin D	400 I.U.
Vitamin E	30 I.U.
Thiamin	1.5 mg
Riboflavin	1.7 mg
Niacin	20 mg
Vitamin B_6	2 mg
Vitamin B_{12}	6 mcg
Folic acid	400 mcg
Biotin	0.3 mg
Pantothenic acid	10 mg
Iron	18 mg
Calcium	1,000 mg
Magnesium	400 mg
Phosphorus	1,000 mg
Iodine	150 mcg
Zinc	15 mg
Copper	2 mg

Endnotes...

INTRODUCTION

1. National Cancer Institute Position Statement, 1998. (www.nci.nih.gov)

2. American Heart Association (AHA) Position Statement, 1998. (www.americanheart.org)

3. Marlett JA. Sites and mechanisms for the hypocholesterolemic actions of soluble dietary fiber sources. In: Kritchevsky D, Bonfield C, eds. *Dietary Fiber in Health and Disease.* New York, NY: Plenum Press, 1997:109–21. Giovannucci E et al. Intake of fat, meat and fiber in relation to risk of colon cancer in men. *Cancer Research* 1994;54:2390–97. Position of the American Dietetic Association: Health implications of dietary fiber. *Journal of the American Dietetic Association* 1997;97:1157–59.

4. Block G et al. Fruit, vegetables and cancer prevention: A review of the epidemiological evidence. *Nutrition and Cancer* 1992;18:1–29. Ness AR et al. Fruit and vegetables, and cardiovascular disease: A review. *International Journal of Epidemiology* 1997;26:1–13. Law MR et al. By how much does fruit and vegetable consumption reduce the risk of ischaemic heart disease? *European Journal of Clinical Nutrition* 1998;52:549–56.

5. Block, 1992. Waladkhani AR et al. Effect of dietary phytochemicals on cancer development. *International Journal of Molecular Medicine* 1998;1:747–53. Goldberg I, ed. *Functional Foods, Designer Foods, Pharmafoods, Nutraceuticals.* New York, NY: Chapman & Hall, 1994.

6. Locksmith GJ et al. Preventing neural tube defects: The importance of periconceptional folic acid supplements. *Obstetrics and Gynecology* 1998;91: 1027–34.

7. Kelly GS. Folates: Supplemental forms and therapeutic applications. *Alternative Medicine Review* 1998;3:208–20. Rimm EG. Folate and vitamin B_6 from diet and supplements in relation to risk for coronary heart disease among women. *Journal of the American Medical Association* 1998;279:349–354. Simons-Morton DG et al. Diet and blood pressure in children and adolescents. *Pediatric Nephrology* 1997;11:244–49.

8. Reid IR. The roles of calcium and vitamin D in the prevention of osteoporosis. *Endocrinology and Metabolism Clinics of North America* 1998;27:389–98.

9. Kotchen TA et al. Dietary sodium and blood pressure: Interactions with other nutrients. *American Journal of Clinical Nutrition* 1997;65(2 suppl):708S–711S.

10. Johnson SR. Premenstrual syndrome therapy. *Clinical Obstetrics and Gynecology* 1998;41:405–21.

11. Levine M et al. Criteria and recommendations for vitamin C intake. *Journal of the American Medical Association* 1999;281:1415–23.

12. Lea MA. Organosulfur compounds and cancer. *Advances in Experimental Medicine and Biology* 1996;401:147–54. Agarwal KC. Therapeutic actions of garlic constituents. *Medicinal Research Reviews* 1996;16:111–24.

13. Anthony MS et al. Effects of soy isoflavones on atherosclerosis: Potential mechanisms. *American Journal of Clinical Nutrition* 1998;68:1390S–93S.

14. Shapiro TA et al. Human metabolism and excretion of cancer chemoprotective glucosinolates and isothiocyanates of cruciferous vegetables. *Cancer Epidemiology, Biomarkers and Prevention* 1998;7:1091–100. Deng XS et al. Prevention of oxidative DNA damage in rats by brussels sprouts. *Free Radical Research* 1998;28:323–33.

15. Sommerburg O et al. Fruits and vegetables that are sources for lutein and zeaxanthin: The macular pigment in human eyes. *British Journal of Ophthalmology* 1998;82:907–10.

16. Clinton SK. Lycopene: Chemistry, biology, and implications for human health and disease. *Nutrition Reviews* 1998;56:35–51. Giovannucci E. Tomatoes, tomato-based products, lycopene, and cancer: Review of the epidemiologic literature. *Journal of the National Cancer Institute* 1999;91:317–31.

17. Frankel EN at al. Inhibition of oxidation of human low-density lipoprotein by phenolic substances in red wine. *The Lancet* 1993;341:454–57. Fuhrman B et al. Consumption of red wine with meals reduces the susceptibility of human plasma and low-density lipoprotein to lipid peroxidation. *American Journal of Clinical Nutrition* 1995;61:549–54.

18. Jang M et al. Cancer chemopreventive activity of reservatrol, a natural product derived from grapes. *Science* 1997;275:218–20. Clement MV et al. Chemopreventive agent reservatrol, a natural product derived from grapes, triggers CD95 signaling-dependent apoptosis in human tumor cells. *Blood* 1998;92:996–1002.

19. Krebs-Smith SM. Progress in improving diet to reduce cancer risk. *Cancer* 1998;85:1425.

20. American Dietetic Association, Press release. 2/23/99.

21. The diet quality of Americans: Strong link with nutrition knowledge. USDA Center for Nutrition Policy and Promotion. August 1998.

22. Krebs-Smith, 1998.

23. Duyff RL. *American Dietetic Association's Complete Food and Nutrition Guide.* Minneapolis, MN: Chronimed Publishing, 1996:144.

24. Is total fat consumption really decreasing? USDA Center for Nutrition Policy and Promotion. April 1998.

25. Dietary guidelines for healthy American adults: A statement for health professionals from the Nutrition Committee, American Heart Association. 1998.

26. U.S. Department of Agriculture Center for Nutrition Policy and Promotion. Dietary guidelines on sodium: Should we take it with a grain of salt? May 1997.

27. U.S. Department of Agriculture Center for Nutrition Policy and Promotion. Is total fat consumption really decreasing? April 1998.

28. U.S. Department of Agriculture. Human Nutrition, ARS Quarterly Report, April–June 1997.

29. Department of Health Services (DHS). 1997 California Dietary Practice Survey.

30. Rimm EB et al. Vitamin E consumption and the risk of coronary disease in men. *New England Journal of Medicine* 1993;328:1450–56. Stampfer MJ et al. Vitamin E consumption and the risk of coronary disease in women. *New England Journal of Medicine* 1993;328:1444–49. Sano M et al. A controlled trial of selegiline, alpha-tocopherol or both as treatment for Alzheimer's disease. The Alzheimer's disease cooperative study. *New England Journal of Medicine* 1997;336:1216–22.

31. The Alpha-Tocopherol, Beta-Carotene Cancer Prevention Study Group. The effect of vitamin E and beta-carotene on the incidence of lung cancer and other cancers in male smokers. *New England Journal of Medicine* 1994; 330:1029–35.

32. Toma S et al. Effectiveness of beta-carotene in cancer chemoprevention. *European Journal of Cancer Prevention* 1995;4:213–24. Hercberg S et al. A primary prevention trial using nutritional doses of antioxidant vitamins and minerals in cardiovascular diseases and cancers in a general population: The SU.VI.MAX study—design, methods, and participant characteristics. SUpplementation en VItamines et Mineraux AntioXydants. *Controlled Clinical Trials* 1998;19:336–51.

33. Tufts University. Modified food guide pyramid for people over seventy years of age, 1999.

34. Hoffman J, Westerdahl J. *Hunza: Secrets of the World's Healthiest and Oldest Living People*. Sacramento, CA: New Wind Publishing, 1997.

35. Eaton SB et al. Stone agers in the fast lane: Chronic degenerative diseases in evolutionary perspective. *American Journal of Medicine* 1988;84:739–49.

36. Barzilai N et al. Revisiting the role of fat mass in the life extension induced by caloric restrictions. *Journal of Gerontology. Series A, Biological Sciences and Medical Sciences* 1999;54:B89–B96. Walford RL et al. Caloric restriction and aging as viewed from Biosphere 2. *Receptor* 1995;5:29–33.

37. Beilin LJ. Vegetarian and other complex diets, fats, fiber, and hypertension. *American Journal of Clinical Nutrition* 1994;59(5 suppl):S1130–S35.

38. Thorogood M et al. Risk of death from cancer and ischaemic heart disease in meat and non-meat eaters. *British Medical Journal* 1994;308:1667–70.

39. Fraser GE et al. Effect of risk factor values on lifetime risk of and age at first coronary event. The Adventist Health Study. *American Journal of Epidemiology* 1995;142:746–58.

40. Diplock AT et al. Functional food science and defence against reactive oxidative species. *British Journal of Nutrition* 1998;80(1 suppl):S77–S112. Lee IM. Antioxidant vitamins in the prevention of cancer. *Proceedings of the Association of American Physicians* 1999;111:10–15.

41. Weisburger JH. Nutritional approach to cancer prevention with emphasis on vitamins, antioxidants, and caretonoids. *American Journal of Clinical Nutrition* 1991;53(1 suppl):226S–37S.

VEGETABLES

1. University of Illinois Department of Food and Science and Human Nutrition. Nutrient conservation in canned, frozen, and fresh foods. October 1997. (www.aces.uiuc.edu/~nutrican/studyfinal.html)

2. Potter JD et al. Vegetables, fruit and phytoestrogens as preventive agents. *IARC Scientific Publications* 1996;139:61–90. Shapiro TA et al. Human metabolism and excretion of cancer chemoprotective glucosinolates and isothiocyanates of cruciferous vegetables. *Cancer Epidemiology, Biomarkers and Prevention* 1998;7:1091–100. Deng XS et al. Prevention of oxidative DNA damage in rats by brussels sprouts. *Free Radical Research* 1998;28: 323–33.

3. Sambaiah K et al. Hypercholesterolemic effect of red bell pepper and capsaicin. *Indian Journal of Experimental Biology* 1980;18:898–99.

4. Mowrey, 1992. Mowrey D. *The Scientific Validation of Herbal Medicine*. New York, NY: Cormorant Books, 1992.

5. Verhoef P et al. Folate and coronary heart disease. *Current Opinion in Lipidology* 1998;9:17–22. Rimm EG. Folate and vitamin B_6 from diet and supplements in relation to risk for coronary heart disease among women. *Journal of the American Medical Association* 1998;279:349–54.

6. Locksmith GJ et al. Preventing neural tube defects: The importance of periconceptional folic acid supplements. *Obstetrics and Gynecology* 1998;91:1027–34. Kelly GS. Folates: Supplemental forms and therapeutic applications. *Alternative Medicine Review* 1998;3:208–20.

7. Sommerburg O et al. Fruits and vegetables that are sources for lutein and zeaxanthin: The macular pigment in human eyes. *British Journal of Ophthalmology* 1998;82:907–10.

8. Breene WM. Nutritional and medicinal value of specialty mushrooms. *Journal of Food Protection* 1990;53:883–89.

9. Potter, 1996.

10. Fukushima S et al. Cancer prevention by organosulfur compounds from garlic and onion. *Journal of Cellular Biochemistry* 1997;27:100–05. Agarwal KC. Therapeutic actions of garlic constituents. *Medicinal Research Reviews* 1996;16:111–24. Argiles JM et al. Prevention of cancer and cardiovascular diseases: A common strategy? *Medicinal Research Reviews* 1998;18:139–48. Berthold HK et al. Effect of a garlic oil preparation on serum lipoproteins and cholesterol metabolism. *Journal of the American Medical Association* 1998;279:1900–02. Isaacsohn JL et al. Garlic powder and plasma lipids and lipoproteins. *Archives of Internal Medicine* 1998;158:1189–94.

11. Hopewell R et al. Soluble fiber: Effect on carbohydrate and lipid metabolism. *Progress in Food and Nutrition Science* 1993;17:159–82. Coats AJ. The potential role of soluble fibre in the treatment of hypercholesterolaemia. *Postgraduate Medical Journal* 1998;74:391–94.

12. Fiber: Still the right choice. *The University of California at Berkeley Wellness Letter* 1999;15:1–2.

13. Wolk A et al. Long-term dietary intake of dietary fiber and decreased risk of coronary heart disease among women. *Journal of the American Medical Association* 1999;281:1998–2004.

14. Wursch P et al. The role of viscous soluble fiber in the metabolic control of diabetes. *Diabetes Care* 1997;20:1774–80.

15. Howe GR et al. Dietary factors and risk of breast cancer: Combined analysis of 12 case-control studies. *Journal of the National Cancer Institute* 1990;82:561–69.

16. Gerber M. Fibre and breast cancer. *European Journal of Cancer Prevention* May 1998;(suppl 2):S63–S67.

17. Rohan TE et al. Dietary factors and the risk of prostate cancer: A case-control study in Ontario, Canada. *Cancer Causes and Control* 1995;6:145–54.

18. Faivre J et al. Primary prevention of colorectal cancer through fibre supplementation. *European Journal of Cancer Prevention* May 1998;(suppl 2):S29–S32.

19. Fuchs CS et al. Dietary fiber and the risk of colorectal cancer and adenoma in women. *New England Journal of Medicine* 1999;340:169–76.

20. Hopewell, 1993.

21. Frohlich RH et al. Cancer preventive value of natural, non–nutritive food constituents. *Acta Medica Austriaca* 1997;24:108–13.

22. Breene, 1990. Chrisan EV, Sands A. Nutritional Value. In Chang ST, Ayes A, eds. *The Biology and Cultivation of Edible Fungi*. New York, NY: Academic Press, 1978.

23. Chang R. Functional properties of edible mushrooms. *Nutrition Reviews* 1996;54(11 pt 2):S91–S93.

24. Chang 1996.

25. Nanba H. Anti-tumor activity of orally administered D-fraction from maitake mushroom. *Journal of Naturopathic Medicine* 1992;4:1–15.

26. Lee WH et al. The Medicinal Benefits of Mushrooms. New Canaan, CN: Keats Publishing, 1985:168.

27. Lee, 1985.

28. Lee, 1985.

29. Lee, 1985.

30. Lee, 1985.

31. U.S.Department of Agriculture. National Organic Program Proposed Rule. February 1995 (www.ams.usda.gov:80/nop/rule/Resource Material Files/labels.pdf)

FRUITS

1. Hopewell R et al. Soluble fiber: Effect on carbohydrate and lipid metabolism. *Progress in Food and Nutrition Science* 1993;17:159–82.

2. Lairon D. Soluble fibers and dietary lipids. *Advances in Experimental Medicine and Biology* 1997;427:99–108.

3. Ness AR, Powles JW. Fruit and vegetables, and cardiovascular disease: A review. *International Journal of Epidemiology* 1997;26:1–13.

4. Steinmetz KA, Potter JD. Vegetables, fruit, and cancer prevention: A review. *Journal of the American Dietetic Association* 1996;96:1027–39.

5. Ziegler RG. Vegetables, fruits, and carotenoids and the risk of cancer. *American Journal of Clinical Nutrition* 1991;53(1 suppl):251S–59S.

6. Potter JD, Steinmetz K. Vegetables, fruit and phytoestrogens as preventive agents. *IARC Scientific Publications* 1996;139:61–90.

7. Duyff RL. *The American Dietetic Association's Complete Food & Nutrition Guide*. Minneapolis, MN: Chronimed Publishing, 1996:86–91.

8. U.S. Department of Agriculture Nutrient Database for Standard Reference. (www.nal.usda.gov/fnic)

9. Fauconneau B et al. Comparative study of radical scavenger and antioxidant properties of phenolic compounds from *Vitis vinifera* cell cultures using in vitro tests. *Life Sciences* 1997;61:2103–10.

10. Miyagi Y et al. Inhibition of human low-density lipoprotein oxidation by flavonoids in red wine and grape juice. *American Journal of Cardiology* 1997;80:1627–31. Osman HE et al. Grape juice but not orange juice or grapefruit juice inhibits platelet activity in dogs and monkeys. *Journal of Nutrition* 1998;128:2307–12.

11. Jang M et al. Cancer chemopreventive activity of reservatrol, a natural product derived from grapes. *Science* 1997;275:218–20. Clement MV et al. Chemopreventive agent reservatrol, a natural product derived from grapes, triggers CD95 signaling-dependent apoptosis in human tumor cells. *Blood* 1998;92:996–1002.

12. Kuzminski LN. Cranberry juice and urinary tract infection: Is there a beneficial relationship? *Nutrition Reviews* 1996;54:S87–S90. Avorn J et al. Reduction of bacteriuria and pyuria after ingestion of cranberry juice. *Journal of the American Medical Association* 1994;271:751–54.

13. Law MR et al. By how much does fruit and vegetable consumption reduce the risk of ischaemic heart disease? *European Journal of Clinical Nutrition* 1998;52:549–56.

14. Giovannucci E. Tomatoes, tomato-based products, lycopene, and cancer: Review of the epidemiologic literature. *Journal of the National Cancer Institute* 1999;91:317–31.

15. Lycopene. Another good reason to eat tomatoes. *Mayo Clinic Health Letter* September 1998;16(9):7.

16. Sies H et al. Lycopene: Antioxidant and biological effects and its bioavailability in the human. *Proceedings of the Society for Experimental Biology* 1998; 218:121–24.

17. U.S. Department of Agriculture Nutrient Database for Standard Reference. USDA-NCC Carotenoid Database for U.S. Foods—1998. (www.nal.usda.gov/fnic)

18. Bendich A. Clinical importance of beta-carotene. *Perspectives in Applied Nutrition* 1993;1:14–22.

GRAINS

1. Verhoef P et al. Folate and coronary heart disease. *Current Opinion in Lipidology* 1998;9:17–22.

2. Pallauf J, Rimbach G. Nutritional significance of phytic acid and phytase. *Archiv fur Tierernahrung* 1997;50:301–19.

3. Thompson LU et al. Phytic acid and minerals: Effect on early markers of risk for mammary and colon carcinogenesis. *Carcinogenesis* 1991;12:2041–45.

4. Vucenik I et al. IP6 in treatment of liver cancer. I. IP6 inhibits growth and reverses transformed phenotype in HepG2 human liver cancer cell line. *AntiCancer Research* 1998;18:4083–90.

5. Wolk A et al. Long-term dietary intake of dietary fiber and decreased risk of coronary heart disease among women. *Journal of the American Medical Association* 1999;281:1998–2004.

6. Hosig KB et al. Comparison of large bowel function and calcium balance during wheat bran and oat bran consumption. *Cereal Chemistry* 1996;73:392–98.

7. U.S. Department of Agriculture Nutrient Database for Standard Reference. (www.nal.usda.gov/fnic)

8. U.S. Department of Agriculture Nutrient Database for Standard Reference. (www.nal.usda.gov/fnic)

9. Hegenbart S. Sugar in the mornin'. *Food Product Design Magazine* June 1996. (www.foodproductdesign.com)

10. Sampling of selected products.

BREADS

1. Howe GR et al. Dietary factors and risk of breast cancer: Combined analysis of 12 case-control studies. *Journal of the National Cancer Institute* 1990;82:561–69.

2. Gerber M. Fibre and breast cancer. *European Journal of Cancer Prevention* May 7, 1998;(2 suppl):S63–S67. Rohan TE et al. Dietary factors and the risk of prostate cancer: A case-control study in Ontario, Canada. *Cancer Causes and Control* 1995;6:145–154.

3. Faivre J et al. Primary prevention of colorectal cancer through fibre supplementation. *European Journal of Cancer Prevention* May 7, 1998;(2 suppl):S29–S32.

4. Coats AJ. The potential role of soluble fibre in the treatment of hypercholesterolaemia. *Postgraduate Medical Journal* 1998;74:391–94.

5. Johnson IT. Antioxidants and anticarcinogens. *European Journal of Cancer Prevention* 1998;7:S55–62.

6. U.S. Department of Agriculture Nutrient Database for Standard Reference. (www.usda.gov/fnic)

7. Pallauf J, Rimbach G. Nutritional significance of phytic acid and phytase. *Archiv fur Tierernahrung* 1997;50:301–19.

8. Thompson LU et al. Phytic acid and minerals: Effect on early markers of risk for mammary and colon carcinogenesis. *Carcinogenesis* 1991;12:2041–45. Graf E et al. Suppression of colonic cancer by dietary phytic acid. *Nutrition and Cancer* 1993;19:9.

9. Verhoef P et al. Folate and coronary heart disease. *Current Opinion in Lipidology* 1998;9:17–22.

10. Wolters MG et al. A continuous in vitro method for estimation of the bioavailability of minerals and trace elements in foods: Application to breads varying in phytic acid content. *British Journal of Nutrition* 1993;69:849–61.

DAIRY AND EGGS

1. U.S. Department of Agriculture Nutrient Database for Standard Reference. (www.nal.usda.gov/fnic)

2. Deciphering the latest report on trans-fats. *Harvard Health Letter* 1998;23:3. Kritchevsky D. Trans-fatty acids and cardiovascular risk. *Prostoglandines Leukotrienes and Essential Fatty Acids* 1997;57:399–402.

3. Judd JT et al. Effects of margarine compared with those of butter on blood lipid profiles related to cardiovascular disease risk factors in normolipemic adults fed controlled diets. *American Journal of Clinical Nutrition* 1998; 68:768–77. Lichtenstein AH et al. Effects of different forms of dietary hydrogenated fats on serum lipoprotein cholesterol levels. *New England Journal of Medicine* 1999;340:1933–40.

4. U.S. Department of Agriculture Nutrient Database for Standard Reference. (www.nal.usda.gov/fnic)

5. Duyff RL. *The American Dietetic Association's Complete Food & Nutrition Guide.* Minneapolis, MN: Chronimed Publishing, 1996:191.

6. Suarez FL, Savaiano DA. Diet, genetics, and lactose intolerance. *Food Technology* 1997;51:74–76.

7. Puri P et al. Splenic and intestinal lymphocyte proliferation response in mice fed milk or yogurt and challenged with *Salmonella typhimurium. International Journal of Food Sciences and Nutrition* 1996;47:391–98.

8. De Simone C et al. The role of probiotics in the modulation of the immune system in man and in animals. *International Journal of Immunotherapy* 1993;9:23–28.

9. Tamai Y et al. Effects of milk fermented by culturing with various lactic acid bacteria and a yeast on serum cholesterol level in rats. *Journal of Fermentation and Bioengineering* 1996;81:181–82.

10. Boutron MC et al. Calcium, phosphorus, vitamin D, dairy products and colorectal carcinogenesis: A French case-controlled study. *British Journal of Cancer* 1996;74:145–51.

11. Sampling of selected products.

12. Lau EM et al. Nutrition and osteoporosis. *Current Opinion in Rheumatology* 1998;10:368–72.

13. Feskanich D et al. Protein consumption and bone fractures in women. *American Journal of Epidemiology* 1996;143:472–79.

14. Coudray C et al. Effect of soluble or partly soluble fiber supplementation on absorption and balance of calcium, magnesium, iron, and zinc in healthy young men. *European Journal of Clinical Nutrition* 1997;51:375–80.

15. Chanda et al. High-lipid intake is a possible predisposing factor in the development of hypogonadal osteoporosis. *Japanese Journal of Physiology* 1996;46:383–88.

16. Duyff RL, 1996.

17. Aro A et al. Stearic acid, trans-fatty acids, and dairy fat: Effects on serum and lipoprotein lipids, apolipoproteins, lipoprotein(a), and lipid transfer proteins in healthy subjects. *American Journal of Clinical Nutrition* 1997;65:1419–26.

18. Schaefer EJ et al. Diet, lipoproteins, and coronary heart disease. *Endocrinology and Metabolism Clinics of North America* 1998;27:711–32, xi.

19. Hu FB et al. A prospective study of egg consumption and risk of cardiovascular disease in men and women. *Journal of the American Medical Association* 1999;281:1387–94.

MEAT AND POULTRY

1. American Heart Association. An eating plan for healthy Americans. 1998. (www.americanheart.org)

2. Macrae FA. Fat and calories in colon and breast cancer: From animal studies to controlled clinical trials. *Preventive Medicine* 1993;22:750–66. Willett WC. Dietary fat intake and cancer risk: A controversial and instructive story. *Seminars in Cancer Biology* 1998;8:245–53. Schaefer EJ, Brousseau ME. Diet, lipoproteins, and coronary heart disease. *Endocrinology and Metabolism Clinics of North America* 1998;27:711–32, xi.

3. Smith KE et al. Quinolone-resistant *Campylobacter jejuni* infections in Minnesota, 1992–1998. *New England Journal of Medicine* 1999; 340:1525–32.

4. Lichtenstein AH et al. Dietary fat consumption and health. *Nutrition Reviews* 1998;56(5 Pt 2):S3–S19, discussion S19–S28.

5. Munoz de Chavez M, Chavez A. Diet that prevents cancer: Recommendations from the American Institute for Cancer Research. *International Journal of Cancer* 1998;11(suppl):85–89.

6. Duyff RL. *The American Dietetic Association's Complete Food & Nutrition Guide.* Minneapolis, MN: Chronimed Publishing, 1996:65.

7. Brown MS, Goldstein JL. A receptor-mediated pathway for cholesterol homeostasis. *Science* 1986;232:34–47. Hegsted DM et al. Dietary fat and serum lipids: An evaluation of the experimental data. *American Journal of Clinical Nutrition* 1993;57:875–83. Skog KI et al. Carcinogenic heterocyclic amines in model systems and cooked foods: A review on formation, occurrence and intake. *Food and Chemical Toxicology* 1998;36:879–96.

8. Fackelman K. Health groups find consensus on fat in diet. *Science News* 1990;137:132.

9. American Heart Association, 1998. (www.americanheart.org)

10. Adapted from U.S. Department of Agriculture Handbook 8-5 and research conducted by Safeway in cooperation with the USDA.

11. Adapted from U.S. Department of Agriculture Handbook 8-5 and research conducted by Safeway in cooperation with the USDA.

12. Hill S. Treatment of nephrotic adults with a supplemented, very low-protein diet. *American Journal of Kidney Diseases* 1996;28:354–64.

13. Environmental Health Information Service. National Toxicology Program, 1998 Report on Carcinogens. 8th ed. (Can be viewed at www.ntp-server.niehs.nih.gov)

14. National Research Council. The Use of Drugs in Food Animals: Benefits and Risks. Washington, D.C.: National Academy Press, 1999.

15. National Research Council, 1999.

16. Zheng W et al. Well-done meat intake and the risk of breast cancer. *Journal of the National Cancer Institute* 1998;90:1724–29.

17. Abdulkarim GB, Smith JS. Heterocyclic amines in fresh and processed meat products. *Journal of Agricultural and Food Chemistry* 1998;46:4680–87.

18. American Institute for Cancer Research. Marinades may drastically decrease cancer risk posed by grilling (press release). 6/18/99.

19. Lappe M. *Mad about Beef.* Gualala, CA: Center for Ethics and Toxics, 1997.

20. Josephson J. Is BSE a threat to human health? *Environmental Health Perspectives* 1998;106:3.

21. U.S. Federal Drug Administration, Center for Veterinary Medicine. Bovine Spongiform Encephalopathy and Cruetzfeldt-Jakob Disease. 1/2/97. (www.fda.gov/cvm/fda/infores/updates/bse/bsefact.html)

22. Centers for Disease Control and Prevention. Bovine Spongiform Encephalopathy (BSE) in the United Kingdom and Creutzfeldt Jakob Disease (CJD) in the United States. (www.cdc.gov/ncidod/diseases)

23. Tan L et al. Risk of transmission of bovine spongiform encephalopathy in the United States. Journal of the American Medical Association 1999;281:2330–39.

24. U.S. Department of Agriculture Nutrient Database for Standard Reference. (www.nal.usda.gov/fnic). California Ostrich Farms. (www.calostrich.com)

FISH AND SEAFOOD

1. Cukier C et al. Biological activity of fish oil. *Arquivos Gastroenterologia* 1996;33:173–78.

2. Stone NJ. Fish consumption, fish oil, lipids, and coronary heart disease. Medical/Scientific Statement, American Heart Association. 1996.

3. Albert CA et al. Fish consumption and risk of sudden cardiac death. *Journal of the American Medical Association* 1998;279:23–28.

4. U. S. Food and Drug Administration. Center for Food Safety and Applied Nutrition, Office of Seafood Handout. 1997.

5. U.S. Department of Agriculture Nutrient Database for Standard Reference. (www.nal.usda.gov/fnic)

6. De Oliveira e Silva ER et al. Effects of shrimp consumption on plasma lipoproteins. *American Journal of Clinical Nutrition* 1996;64:712–17.

7. Simopoulos AP. Omega-3 fatty acids in health and disease and in growth and development. *American Journal of Clinical Nutrition* 1991;54:438–63.

8. Connor WE et al. N-3 fatty acids from fish oil: effects on plasma lipoproteins and hypertriglyceridemic patients. *Annals of the New York Academy of Sciences* 1993;638:16–34.

9. Simopoulos AP. Omega-3 fatty acids in the prevention-management of cardiovascular disease. *Canadian Journal of Physiology and Pharmacology* 1997;75:234–39.

10. Albert CA et al, 1998.

11. Ariza-Ariza R et al. Omega-3 fatty acids in rheumatoid arthritis: An overview. *Seminars in Arthritis and Rheumatism* 1998;27:366–70.

12. U.S. Food and Drug Administration. Center for Food Safety and Applied Nutrition. (vm.cfsan.fda.gov/index.html)

13. Mirvish SS et al. Effect of ascorbic acid dose taken with a meal in nitrosoproline excretion in subjects ingesting nitrate and proline. *Nutrition and Cancer* 1998;31:106–10. Xu GP et al. Effects of fruit juices, processed vegetable juice, orange peel and green tea on endogenous formation of N-nitrosoproline in subjects from a high-risk area for gastric cancer in Moping County, China. *European Journal of Cancer Prevention* 1993;4:327–35.

14. Fish Consumption Advisory, Minnesota Department of Natural Resources, 1998.

LEGUMES

1. Hopewell R et al. Soluble fiber: Effect on carbohydrate and lipid metabolism. *Progress in Food and Nutrition Science* 1993;17:159–82.

2. Shinnick FL et al. Serum cholesterol reduction by oats and other fiber sources. *Cereal Foods World* 1991;36:815–21.

3. Lairon D. Soluble fibers and dietary lipids. *Advances in Experimental Medicine and Biology* 1997;427:99–108.

4. Rimm EG. Folate and vitamin B_6 from diet and supplements in relation to risk for coronary heart disease among women. *Journal of the American Medical Association* 1998;279:349–54. McCully KS. Homocysteine, folate, vitamin B_6 and cardiovascular disease (editorial). *Journal of the American Medical Association* 1998;279:392–93.

5. Fournier DB et al. Soy, its components, and cancer prevention: A review of the in vitro, animal, and human data. *Cancer Epidemiology, Biomarkers and Prevention* 1998;7:1055–65.

6. Potter JD et al. Vegetables, fruit and phytoestrogens as preventive agents. *IARC Scientific Publications* 1996;139:61–90.

7. U.S. Department of Agriculture Food and Nutrition Information Center. (www.nal.usda.gov/fnic)

8. Knight DC et al. A review of the clinical effects of phytoestrogens. *Obstetrics and Gynecology* 1996;87(5 Pt 2):897–904.

9. Lichenstein AH. Soy protein, isoflavones and cardiovascular disease risk. *Journal of Nutrition* 1998;128:1589–92.

10. Messina MJ et al. Soy intake and cancer risk: A review of the in vitro and in vivo data. *Nutrition and Cancer* 1994;21:113–31.

11. Stoll BA. Eating to beat breast cancer: Potential role for soy supplements. *Annals of Oncology* 1997;8:223–25.

12. Wong WW et al. Cholesterol-lowering effect of soy protein in normocholesterolemic and hypercholesterolemic men. *American Journal of Clinical Nutrition* 1998;68(6 suppl):1385S–89S.

13. Brandi ML. Natural and synthetic isoflavones in the prevention and treatment of chronic diseases. *Calcified Tissue International* 1997;61 (1 suppl):S5–S8.

14. Clarkson TB et al. The potential of soybean phytoestrogens for postmenopausal hormone replacement therapy. *Proceedings of the Society for Experimental Biology* 1998;217:365–68.

15. Miyagi Y et al. Trypsin inhibitor activity in commercial soybean products in Japan. *Journal of Nutrition Science Vitaminology* 1997;43:575–80.

16. Liener IE. Possible adverse effects of soybean. *Journal of Nutrition* 1995;125(3 suppl):744S–50S.

17. Divi RL et al. Anti-thyroid isoflavones from soybean: Isolation, characterization, and mechanisms of action. *Biochemical Pharmacology* 1997;54:1087–96.

18. Setchell KD et al. Dietary estrogens—a probable cause of infertility and liver disease in captive cheetahs. *Gastroenterology* 1987;93:225–33.

19. Irvine CH et al. Phytoestrogens in soy-based infant foods: Concentrations, daily intake, and possible biological effects. *Proceedings of the Society for Experimental Biology* 1998;217:247–53.

NUTS AND SEEDS

1. U.S.Department of Agriculture Nutrient Database for Standard Reference. (www.nal.usda.gov/fnic)

2. Tham DM et al. Potential health benefits of dietary phytoestrogens: A review of the clinical, epidemiological, and mechanistic evidence. *Journal of Clinical Endocrinology and Metabolism* 1998;83:2223–35.

3. Rozanova IA et al. Effect of antiatherosclerotic diet, containing polyunsaturated fatty acids of the omega-3 family from flax oil, on fatty acid composition of cell membranes of patients with ischemic heart disease. Hypertensive disease and hyperlipoproteinemia. *Voprosy Pitaniia* 1997;5:15–17.

4. Tham DM et al. Clinical review 97: Potential health benefits of dietary phytoestrogens: A review of the clinical, epidemiological, and mechanistic evidence. *Journal of Clinical Endocrinology and Metabolism* 1998;83:2223–35.

5. Hennekens C, Stampfer M. The Physician's Health Study. *New England Journal of Medicine* 1989;321:183–85, 129–35.

6. Sabate J et al. Effects of walnuts on serum lipid levels and blood pressure in normal men. *New England Journal of Medicine* 1993;328:603–07.

7. Ip C, Lisk DJ. Bioactivity of selenium from Brazil nut for cancer prevention and selenoenzyme maintenance. *Nutrition and Cancer* 1994;21:203–12.

8. Spiller GA et al. Nuts and plasma lipids: An almond-based diet lowers LDL-C while preserving HDL-C. *Journal of the American College of Nutrition* 1998;17:285–90.

9. Abbey M et al. Partial replacement of saturated fatty acids with almonds or walnuts lowers total plasma cholesterol and low-density-lipoprotein cholesterol. *American Journal of Clinical Nutrition* 1994;59:995–99.

10. Bracher F. Phytotherapy of benign prostatic hyperplasia. *Urologe. Ausgabe.* 1997;36:10–17.

11. Lee L. *The Enzyme Cure.* Tiburon, CA: Future Medicine Publishing, 1998: 54–55.

12. U.S. Department of Agriculture Nutrient Database for Standard Reference. (www.nal.usda.gov/fnic)

VEGETARIAN ALTERNATIVES

1. 1997 Vegetarian Resource Group-sponsored Roper Poll.

2. Jacob RA, Burri BJ. Oxidative damage and defense. *American Journal of Clinical Nutrition* 1996;63(suppl):985S–90S.

3. Knutsen SF. Lifestyle and the use of health services. *American Journal of Clinical Nutrition* 1994;59(5 suppl):1171S–75S.

4. Key TH et al. Dietary habits and mortality in 11,000 vegetarian and health conscious people: Results of a 17-year follow up. *British Medical Journal* 1996;313:775–79.

5. Beilin LJ. Vegetarian and other complex diets, fats, fiber, and hypertension. *American Journal of Clinical Nutrition* 1994;59(5 suppl):1130–35.

6. Dwyer JT. Health aspects of vegetarian diets. *American Journal of Clinical Nutrition* 1988;48(3 suppl):712–738.

7. Thorogood M et al. Risk of death from cancer and ischaemic heart disease in meat and non-meat eaters. *British Medical Journal* 1994;308:1667–70.

8. Franklin TL et al. Adherence to very low fat diet by a group of cardiac rehabilitation patients in the rural southeastern United States. *Archives of Family Medicine* 1995;4:551–54.

9. Ornish D et al. Intensive lifestyle changes for reversal of coronary heart disease. *Journal of the American Medical Association* 1998;280:2001–07.

10. Mills PK et al. Cancer incidence among California Seventh-day Adventists, 1976–1982. *American Journal of Clinical Nutrition* 1994;59(5 suppl):1136S–42S.

11. Messina MJ, Messina VL. *The Dietitian's Guide to Vegetarian Diets: Issues and Applications.* Gaithersburg, MD: Aspen Publishers, 1996.

12. Young VR, Pellett PL. Plant proteins in relation to human protein and amino acid nutrition. *American Journal of Clinical Nutrition* 1994;59 (5 suppl):1203S–12S.

13. U.S. Department of Agriculture. Food and Nutrient Intakes by Region, 1994–96. (www.barc.usda.gov/bhnrc/foodsurvey)

14. Slatter ML et al. Meat consumption and its association with other diet and health factors in young adults: The CARDIA study. *American Journal of Clinical Nutrition* 1992;56:699–704.

15. Tesar R et al. Axial and peripheral bone density and nutrient intakes of postmenopausal vegetarian and omnivorous women. *American Journal of Clinical Nutrition* 1992;56:699–704.

16. Remer T, Manz F. Estimation of the renal net acid excretion by adults consuming diets containing variable amounts of protein. *American Journal of Clinical Nutrition* 1994; 59:1356–1361.

17. Germano C. *The Osteoporosis Solution.* New York, NY: Kensington Books, 1998.

18. Weaver CM, Plawecki KL. Dietary calcium: Adequacy of a vegetarian diet. *American Journal of Clinical Nutrition* 1994;59(suppl):1238S–41S.

19. Helman AD, Darnton-Hill I. Vitamin and iron status in new vegetarians. *American Journal of Clinical Nutrition* 1987;45:785–89.

20. Craig WJ. Iron status of vegetarians. *American Journal of Clinical Nutrition* 1994;59(5 suppl):1233S–37S.

21. Herbert V. Vitamin B_{12}: Plant sources, requirements, and assay. *American Journal of Clinical Nutrition* 1988;48:852–58.

22. Helman AD, Darnton-Hill I. Vitamin and iron status in new vegetarians. *American Journal of Clinical Nutrition* 1987;45:785–89.

23. Henderson JB et al. The importance of limited exposure to ultraviolet radiation and dietary factors in the aetiology of Asian rickets: A risk-factor model. *Quarterly Journal of Nutrition* 1987;63:413–25.

24. Holick MF. Vitamin D and bone health. *Journal of Nutrition* 1996;126 (4 suppl):1159S–64S.

25. Sanders TAB, Roshanai F. Platelet phospholipid fatty acid composition and function in vegans compared with age-and sex-matched omnivore controls. *European Journal of Clinical Nutrition* 1992;46:823–31.

26. Conquer JA, Holub BJ. Dietary docosahexaenoic acid as a source of eicosapentaenoic acid in vegetarians and omnivores. *Lipids* 1997;32:341–45.

27. Freeland-Graves JH et al. Zinc status of vegetarians. *Journal of the American Dietetic Association* 1980;77:655–61.

28. Food and Nutrition Board, National Academy of Sciences—National Research Council. *Recommended Dietary Allowances: 10th Edition* (Revised 1989). Washington, D.C.: National Academy Press, 1999.

29. Sampling of selected products.

30. Sampling of selected products.

FATS AND OILS

1. Stoll BA. Association between breast and colorectal cancers. *British Journal of Surgery* 1998;85:1468–72.

2. Masley SC. Dietary therapy for preventing and treating coronary artery disease. *American Family Physician* 1998;57:1299–1306, 1307–09.

3. de Lorgeril M et al. Mediterranean diet, traditional risk factors, and the rate of cardiovascular complications after myocardial infarction. *Circulation* 1999;99:779–85. Leaf A. Dietary prevention of coronary heart disease: The Lyon Diet Heart Study. *Circulation* 1999;99:733–35.

4. Wolk A et al. A prospective study of association of monounsaturated fat and other types of fat with risk of breast cancer. *Archives of Internal Medicine* 1998;158:41–45.

5. Simopoulos AP. Omega-3 fatty acids in health and disease and in growth and development. *American Journal of Clinical Nutrition* 1991;54:438–63.

6. Deciphering the latest report on trans-fats. *Harvard Health Letter* 1998;23:3. Kritchevsky D. Trans-fatty acids and cardiovascular risk. *Prostoglandins Leukotrienes and Essential Fatty Acids* 1997;57:399–402. Pedersen JI et al. Trans-fatty acids and health. *Tidsskrift for den Norske Laegeforening* 1998 20;118:3474–80.

7. Lichtenstein AH et al. Effects of different forms of dietary hydrogenated fats on serum lipoprotein cholesterol levels. *New England Journal of Medicine* 1999;340:1933–40.

8. Simopoulos, 1991.

9. Leaf, 1999.

10. Noguchi M et al. The role of fatty acids and eicosanoid synthesis inhibitors in breast carcinoma. *Oncology* 1995;52:265–71.

11. Zock PL et al. Linoleic acid intake and cancer risk: A review and meta-analysis. *American Journal of Clinical Nutrition* 1998;68:142–53.

12. Wolk A et al, 1998.

13. Storlien LH et al. Dietary fats and insulin action. *Diabetologia* 1996 39:621–31. Storlien LH et al. Skeletal muscle membrane lipids and insulin resistance. *Lipids* March 1996;(suppl):S261–S65.

14. Munoz de Chavez M, Chavez A. Diet that prevents cancer: Recommendations from the American Institute for Cancer Research. *International Journal of Cancer* 1998;11(suppl):85–89.

15. Brown MS, Goldstein JL. A receptor-mediated pathway for cholesterol homeostasis. *Science* 1986;232:34–47. Hegsted DM et al. Dietary fat and serum lipids: An evaluation of the experimental data. *American Journal of Clinical Nutrition* 1993;57:875–83. Skog KI et al. Carcinogenic heterocyclic amines in model systems and cooked foods: A review on formation, occurrence and intake. *Food and Chemical Toxicology* 1998;36:879–96.

16. Pahor M et al. Emerging noninvasive biochemical measures to predict cardiovascular risk. *Archives of Internal Medicine* 1999;159:237–45.

17. American Heart Association. (www.americanheart.org)

18. Oliver MF. It is more important to increase the intake of unsaturated fats than to decrease the intake of saturated fats: Evidence from clinical trials relating to ischemic heart disease. *American Journal of Clinical Nutrition* 1997;66(4 suppl):980S–86S.

19. Ornish D et al. Intensive lifestyle changes for reversal of coronary heart disease. *Journal of the American Medical Association* 1998;280:2001–07.

20. Cheskin LJ et al. Gastrointestinal symptoms following consumption of olestra or regular triglyceride potato chips: A controlled comparison. *Journal of the American Medical Association* 1998;279:150–52.

21. De Graaf C et al. Nonabsorbable fat (sucrose polyester) and the regulation of energy intake and body weight. *American Journal of Physiology* 1996;270:R1386–R93.

22. Blackburn H. Sounding board—olestra and the FDA. *New England Journal of Medicine* 1996;334:984–86.

23. Westrate JA, van het Hof KH. Sucrose polyester and plasma carotenoid concentrations in healthy subjects. *American Journal of Clinical Nutrition* 1995;62:591–97.

HERBS AND SPICES

1. Esslinger KA et al. Dietary sodium intake and mortality. *Nutrition Reviews* 1998;56:311–13.

2. Hirohata T et al. Diet/nutrition and stomach cancer in Japan. *International Journal of Cancer* 1997;10(suppl):34–36.

3. Kushi M. The Macrobiotic Way. Garden City Park, NY: Avery Publishing Group, 1993:72–74.

4. Dietary guidance on sodium: Should we take it with a grain of salt? USDA Center for Nutrition Policy and Promotion. May 1997.

5. Duyff R.D. *The American Dietetic Association's Complete Food & Nutrition Guide.* Minneapolis, MN: Chronimed Publishing, 1996:154–62.

6. Surh YJ et al. Chemoprotective properties of some pungent ingredients present in red pepper and ginger. *Mutation Research* 1998;402:259–67.

7. Matsuda H et al. Anti-inflammatory activity of ginsenoside Ro. *Planta Medica* 1990;56:19–23.

8. Tanaka S et al. Antiulcerogenic compounds isolated from Chinese cinnamon. *Planta Medica* 1989;55:245–48.

9. Shcherbanovsky LR et al. Volatile oil of Anethum Graveolens L. as an inhibitor of yeast and lactic acid bacteria. *Prikladnaia Biokhimiia Mikrobiologiia* 1975;11:476–77.

10. Argiles JM et al. Prevention of cancer and cardiovascular diseases: A common strategy? *Medicinal Research Reviews* 1998;18:139–48.

11. Fukushima S et al. Cancer prevention by organosulfur compounds from garlic and onion. *Journal of Cellular Biochemistry* 1997;27:100–05.

12. Aikins Murphy P. Alternative therapies for nausea and vomiting of pregnancy. *Obstetrics and Gynecology* 1998;91:149–55.

13. Bordia A et al. Effect of ginger (*Zingiber officinale Rosc.*) and fenugreek (*Trigonella foenumgraecum L.*) on blood lipids, blood sugar and platelet aggregation in patients with coronary artery disease. *Prostaglandins, Leukotrienes and Essential Fatty Acids* 1997;58:379–84.

14. Tyler V. *Herbs of Choice.* Binghamton, NY: Haworth Press, 1994:76.

15. Singletary K et al. Inhibition by rosemary and carnosol of 7,12-dimethylbenz[a]anthracene (DMBA)-induced rat mammary tumorigenesis and in vivo DMBA-DNA adduct formation. *Cancer Letters* 1996;104:43–48.

16. Tawfiq N et al. Induction of the anti-carcinogenic enzyme quinone reductase by food extracts using murine hepatoma cells. *European Journal of Cancer Prevention* 1994;3:285–92.

17. Krishnaswamy K. Indian functional foods: Roles in prevention of cancer. *Nutrition Reviews* 1996;54:S127–S131.

SUGARS AND SWEETENERS

1. Position of the American Dietetic Association: Use of nutritive and nonnutritive sweeteners. *Journal of the American Dietetic Association* 1998;98:580–87.

2. Anderson G. Sugars and health: A review. *Nutrition Research* 1997;17:1485–98.

3. U.S. Department of Health and Human Services/National Institutes of Health. National Toxicology Program. Seventh Annual Report on Carcinogens: Saccharin. Washington DC, 1994:CAS No. 128-44-99.

4. U.S. Department of Health and Human Services Health Hazard Evaluation. Summary of Adverse Reactions Attributed to Aspartame. Washington DC, 1995.

5. Position of the American Dietetic Association: Use of nutritive and nonnutritive sweeteners. *Journal of the American Dietetic Association* 1998;98:580–87.

6. Shaywitz B et al. Aspartame, behavior, and cognitive function in children with attention deficit disorders. *Pediatrics* 1994;93:70–75.

7. Olney J et al. Increasing brain tumor rates: Is there a link to aspartame? *Journal of Neuropathology and Experimental Neurology* 1996;55:115–123.

8. *Journal of the American Dietetic Association,* 1998.

9. American Diabetes Association. (www.diabetes.org/nutrition/faqs)

10. *Journal of the American Dietetic Association,* 1998.

DELI

1. U.S. Department of Agriculture Food and Nutrition Information Center, Agricultural Research Service. (www.usda.gov/agency)

2. Lichten JV. *Dining Lean.* Houston, TX: Nutrifit Publishing, 1998:152.

3. U.S. Department of Agriculture Nutrient Database for Standard Reference. (www.usda.gov/fnic) Lichten, 1998.

4. U.S. Department of Agriculture. World Health Statistics Quarterly. August 1998.

5. FDA Center for Food Safety & Applied Nutrition. Foodborne Pathogenic Microorganisms and Natural Toxins Handbook, 1997.

6. Van Beneden CA et al. Multinational outbreak of *Salmonella enterica* serotype newport infections due to contaminated alfalfa sprouts. *Journal of the American Medical Association* 1999;281:158–62.

7. Centers for Disease Control. Federal Register of September 22 (62 FR 49519). September 24, 1997.

PACKAGED FOODS

1. U.S. Department of Agriculture Center for Nutrition Policy and Promotion. Dietary guidance on sodium: Should we take it with a grain of salt? May 1997.

2. Survey of selected products, and U.S. Department of Agriculture Food and Nutrition Information Center. (www.nal.usda.gov/fnic)

3. Earning a slice of the global pie. *Chemical Marketing Reporter* 6/16/97.

4. U.S. Food and Drug Administration. Center For Food Safety. (vm.cfsan.fda.gov/index.html)

5. FDA Center for Food Safety.

6. FDA Center for Food Safety.

7. U.S. Department of Health and Human Services Public Health Service. FDA Talk Paper (Press release). Rockville, MD: Food and Drug Administration, U.S. Department of Health and Human Services Public Health Service, 5/7/97.

8. FDA Center for Food Safety.

9. Variyam JN et al. USDA's Healthy eating index and nutrition information. Food and Rural Economics Division, Economic Research Service, and Center for Nutrition Policy and Promotion, USDA. Technical Bulletin No. 1866. April 1998. (www.econ.ag.gov/epubs/pdf/tb1866)

10. Kristal AR et al. Trends in food label use associated with new nutrition labeling regulations. *American Journal of Public Health* 1998;88:1212–15.

11. U.S. Food and Drug Administration. The Food Label. February 1999. (www.fda.gov/opacom/backgrounders/foodlabel)

12. American Heart Association. Trans-Fatty Acids and Stroke Guide. (www.americanheart.org)

SNACKS

1. Sampling of selected products.

2. Denke MA, Grundy SM. Effects of fats high in stearic acid on lipid and lipoprotein concentrations in men. *American Journal of Clinical Nutrition* 1991;54:1036–40.

3. Osakabe N et al. The antioxidant substances in cacao liquor. *Journal of Nutritional Science and Vitaminology* 1998:44:313–21.

4. Sanbongi C et al. Polyphenols in chocolate, which have antioxidant activity, modulate immune functions in humans in vitro. *Cellular Immunology* 1997;177:129–36.

5. U.S. Department of Agriculture Nutrient Database for Standard Reference. (www.nal.usda.gov/fnic)

6. Sampling of selected products.

7. Tyler V. *Herbs Of Choice*. Binghamton, New York: Haworth Press, 1995:132–34.

8. Survey of selected products, and U.S. Department of Agriculture Nutrient Database for Standard Reference. (www.nal.usda.gov/fnic)

BEVERAGES

1. Kleiner SM. Water: An essential but overlooked nutrient. *Journal of the American Dietetic Association* 1999;99:200–06.

2. Tufts University. Modified Food Guide Pyramid for People over Seventy Years of Age, 1999.

3. Giddings M. The undiluted truth about drinking water. *Guidelines for Canadian Drinking Water Quality* 4/10/97:1–26.

4. Clark S. When it comes to safe drinking water, there's more than meeting the regulations. *Opflow* 1998;24:1–3.

5. National Resources Defense Council. Bottled water: Pure drink or pure hype? Petition to the FDA. March 1999.

6. Halpern GM et al. Comparative uptake of calcium from milk and a calcium-rich mineral water in lactose intolerant adults: Implications for treatment of osteoporosis. *American Journal of Preventive Medicine* 1991;7:379–83.

7. National Resources Defense Council. March 1999.

8. Jacobson MF. Liquid candy: How soft drinks are harming Americans' health. *Nutrition Action Newsletter* (Center for Science in the Public Interest). 10/21/98.

9. Willhite L. Osteoporosis in women: Prevention and treatment. *Journal of the American Pharmaceutical Association* 1998;38:614–23.

10. Jacobson, 1988.

11. National Institute of Environmental Health Sciences. The truth about caffeine. 1997. (www.niehs.nih.gov/odhsb/focus)

12. Robelin M, Rogers PJ. Mood and psychomotor performance effects of the first, but not of subsequent, cup-of-coffee equivalent doses of caffeine consumed after overnight caffeine abstinence. *Behavioural Pharmacology* 1998;9:611–18.

13. Nehlig A. Are we dependent upon coffee and caffeine? A review on human and animal data. *Neuroscience and Biobehavioral Reviews* 1999;23:563–76.

14. Nutt DJ et al. Brain mechanisms of social anxiety disorder. *Journal of Clinical Psychiatry* 1998;59(suppl)17:4–11.

15. Ugarriza DN et al. Premenstrual syndrome: Diagnosis and intervention. *Nurse Practitioner* 1998;23:49–52.

16. Kleiner, 1999.

17. Rollins N et al. Dietary caffeine intake and bone status of postmenopausal women. *American Journal of Clinical Nutrition* 1997;65:1826–30.

18. Lau EM et al. Nutrition and osteoporosis. *Current Opinion in Rheumatology* 1998;10:368–72.

19. O'Connell MB. Prevention and treatment of osteoporosis. *Pharmacotherapy* 1999;19(1 Pt 2):7S–20S.

20. Leitzman F et al. A prospective study of coffee consumption and the risk of symptomatic gallstone disease in men. *Journal of the American Medical Association* 1999;281:2106–12.

21. U.S. Department of Agriculture Nutrient Data for Standard Reference. (www.usda.gov/fnic) Duyff, RL. *The American Dietetic Association's Complete Food and Nutrition Guide.* Minneapolis, MN: Chronimed Publishing, 1996:178.

22. Blot WJ et al. Cancer rates among drinkers of black tea. *Critical Reviews in Food Science and Nutrition* 1997;37:739–60.

23. Bushman JL. Green tea and cancer in humans: A review of the literature. *Nutrition and Cancer* 1998;31:151–59.

24. Hennekens CH. Alcohol and risk of coronary events. *Alcohol and the Cardiovascular System.* Bethesda, MD: National Institutes of Health, 1996:15–24.

25. Fuhrman B et al. Consumption of red wine with meals reduces the susceptibility of human plasma and low-density lipoprotein to lipid peroxidation. *American Journal of Clinical Nutrition* 1995;61:549–54.

26. Frankel EN et al. Inhibition of oxidation of human low density lipoprotein by phenolic substances in red wine. *The Lancet* 1993;341:454–57.

27. Ridker P. Association of moderate alcohol consumption and plasma concentration of endogenous tissue-type plasminogen activator. *Journal of the American Medical Association* 1994;272:929–33.

28. Wannamethee SG, Shaper AG. Type of alcohol drink and risk of major coronary heart disease events and all-cause mortality. *American Journal of Public Health* 1999;899:685–90. Gaziano JM et al. Type of alcoholic beverage and risk of myocardial infarction. *American Journal of Cardiology* 1999;83:52–57.

29. USDA Center for Nutrition Policy and Promotion. Does alcohol have a place in a healthy diet? August 1997.

Index...

Notes

Notes

Notes